Therapi
Emotional \

For Vivienne, sister and seeker of the heart

THIS IS A CARLTON BOOK

Design copyright © 2001, 2003 Carlton Books Limited
Text copyright © 2001 Jane Alexander

This edition published by
Carlton Books Limited 2003
20 Mortimer Street, London W1T 3JW

A CIP catalogue record for this book is available from
the British Library
ISBN 1 84222 884 6

Printed and bound in England

The author of this book is not a physician and the ideas, procedures and suggestions in this
book are intended to supplement, not replace, the medical and legal advice of trained
professionals. All matters regarding your health require medical supervision. Consult your
medical practitioner before adopting the suggestions in this book, as well as about any
condition that may require diagnosis or medical attention.

The authors and the publisher have made every effort to ensure that
all the information in this book is correct and up to date at the time of publication. Neither
the authors nor the publisher can accept responsibility for any accident, injury or damage
that results from using the ideas, information or advice offered in this book.

Therapies for Emotional Wellbeing

A Complete Guide to Holistic Therapies for
Emotional Healing and Spirituality

Jane Alexander

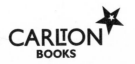

CARLTON
BOOKS

Contents

Introduction

Life is for living, so why aren't you living life to the full? In today's frenetic, stress-filled world, it's all too easy to let life pass you by. Most of us feel life is a struggle: a battle to get fit and healthy, a fight to meet deadlines and pay the bills. Our relationships with our own selves can be less than congenial; our relationships with others are often fraught. Few of us even think about our relationship with the spiritual world – we simply don't have the time.

Yet all the information we need to lead healthier, happier, more fulfilled lives is ours for the taking. The fields of natural healing, mind–body medicine, psychology and spiritual understanding offer many paths to a vital yet peaceful life. Unfortunately we can often become overwhelmed by the sheer choice.

There are literally hundreds of different therapies and teachings all promising to heal your mind, emotions and soul in some way. Which should you choose? Where do you start? The choice can be bewildering. Fortunately, the answers lie within the pages of one book – this one.

The aim of *Therapies for Emotional Wellbeing* is to provide a simple, straightforward, friendly guide through the maze of holistic living. We have done all the hard work for you, picking out the nuggets of sheer gold amid the tomes of heavy theory and complex philosophy. As you work your way through this clear and concise book, you will readily learn how to incorporate emotional healing and spirituality into everyday life. There is no preaching or dictating in these pages; you are merely presented with useful, effective information and techniques that really work. *Therapies for Emotional Wellbeing* offers a manual for twenty-first-century living, a guide to living your life to the full – each and every day.

How to use this book

How you use this book is entirely up to you. There is a lot of information here – probably way too much for any one person to incorporate into their life! You most certainly *can* read it through from start to finish, but I suspect that most people will find they want to dip in and out. That's fine. Most chapters will stand quite happily alone. You can let your intuition do the deciding – flick through the contents and see what grabs your attention. Or, if you really want to let your unconscious mind choose what it needs, close your eyes and flick through the pages until you feel drawn to stop. Open your eyes and see where you've landed. You may well be surprised to find how relevant the page is to you.

Taking responsibility

I firmly believe that the most important thing any of us can do is to take responsibility for our lives. Once we decide that we have the power to change, almost anything can happen.

In the past, it has been common for many of us to hand over responsibility for our emotional wellbeing and spiritual lives to other people: to teachers and therapists; to priests and ministers. We have relied heavily on the opinions and thoughts of other people; we have looked to newspapers, television and society for approval. Yet, when you decide that *you* are in charge of your destiny, it is almost as if a quantum leap occurs and absolutely everything is open to change.

Rest assured, you don't have to go out and make major changes overnight. Even the tiniest shift can create ripples. Practise a ritual, say a prayer and you will have begun a process that almost inevitably leads to other changes. You can develop new ways of living and loving, so that your relationships become more fulfilling and exciting. Work need not be a drag and a duty. Your spirit can be allowed to soar.

When to seek professional help

This book offers plenty of suggestions for leading a happier life. Yet it cannot work miracles. There are times when you will need expert help. Although I have included numerous self-help tips and do-it-yourself techniques, I would strongly recommend that, if you are drawn to a particular therapy or practice, you seek out an experienced, well-qualified practitioner. A large resource section has been supplied at the end of this book, which lists reputable organizations through which you should be able to get in touch with your nearest qualified practitioner (see page 124).

If you feel that your psychological or emotional state is precarious – if, for example, you feel suicidal, are suffering from chronic depression, are psychotic or have severe mental health problems – you need to see an experienced physician or psychiatrist. Also, be aware that many of the exercises in this book are designed to shift emotions and, in the process, they may bring past traumas or difficulties to the surface. If you know that you have painful events in your past, any abuse or trauma for example, it is advisable to work alongside a well-qualified psychotherapist who can help you through any tough times.

Part 1 *Mind and Emotions*

Our minds and emotions play as large a role as our bodies in maintaining health and well-being. Yet few of us think to give ourselves mental and emotional workouts. Nowadays, there is really no excuse for not 'mindworking'. Simple techniques can help you stressproof your life and reduce your levels of tension and anxiety, helping you cope with everyday life.

Meditation has been proven, in numerous studies, to be an incredible stressbuster. If you have never tried it before, now could be the time to give this incredible system a chance. If you have tried it but found it too difficult, mindfulness techniques offer many of the benefits without the hard work, while autogenic training is a tried and trusted formula with a proven track record.

In the past, psychotherapy gained a reputation for being long-winded and intrusive. Many people felt they couldn't justify the time, effort and money required for long-term analysis. Yet new forms of 'talking therapies' offer all manner of variations on the counselling theme. Whatever your disposition, time and finances, there is bound to be something for you – and it is good to talk.

Later in this section, we will look at work – how to escape the feeling that work is drudgery and make it really 'work' for you. We will also look at simple, effective ways to improve your everyday relationships – with friends, family, colleagues. But it isn't all hard work: discovering how to give your sex life a boost has to count as good fun! Meanwhile, boosting your creativity with dance, art and music can be a real eye-opener. Many of us simply don't allow ourselves the time to explore our natural creativity, but it can bring untold benefits.

Finally, our dreams offer a wonderful way of working in the most natural way with our psyches. Dreaming gives us a direct route to the unconscious – it's the way our deep-rooted emotions, fears and anxieties can communicate with our waking, conscious mind. We'll look at ways to work with these messengers of the night.

This section will help you to pinpoint the areas in your life that need attention and offer some interesting solutions and routes to explore. I would never expect you to take everything on board, but hope that you will gain a good idea of what might work for you.

1 Stress

Stress is a fact of life. Whether it be superhuman deadlines at work, the hassle of the morning commute or babies who just won't stop crying, the causes of stress are something few people escape. Yet, according to doctors, stress can be a silent, deadly killer.

Under stress, the body produces the hormones cortisol and adrenaline, which cause changes in heart rate, blood pressure and metabolism to prepare the body for fight or flight. In normal life, we can hardly run away from the office or punch the boss, so the body does not get rid of the excess hormones, resulting in unproductive, or harmful, stress.

Untreated, long-term, continual stress can manifest itself in depression, anxiety, palpitations, ulcers, headaches or irregularities in the menstrual cycle. Allergic reactions can even be triggered by stress. Fortunately, doctors are starting to become more sympathetic towards the problem. Whereas the old tendency was either to dismiss the question entirely or to fob the patient off with tranquillizers, many doctors are now suggesting self-help techniques such as deep breathing and relaxation, hypnotherapy and meditation to teach people how to deal with the condition.

Yet many people feel they have no right to admit to stress, and dismiss the whole idea. They argue that we never used to have all this stress: in the 'old days', we just got on with life and didn't waste time complaining about intangible problems such as stress. Well, it may well seem like that, but do remember that we no longer live in the world of yesteryear. We live in a world that is changing faster than ever before. There are people alive who grew up without air travel, without television, without computers and the Internet, without superstores and convenience foods. Life was totally different. Not that there weren't stressful factors – certainly poverty was far more prevalent and life could be excessively hard – but the sheer speed of life wasn't there. Nowadays, we are all jugglers – balancing home and career in ways our ancestors simply couldn't have envisaged. The causes of modern stress are myriad. But how do you deal with it?

The key to combating stress is realizing what pushes your buttons, what causes you stress. Do you feel stress just on the odd occasion or is your problem more deep-seated?

Coping strategies

Shock tactics for short-term stress

These tactics can be useful for when you need immediate relief from tension and stress.

1 Don't fly to the coffee machine or reach for a Coke – caffeine merely exacerbates your stress responses. Drink a long, cool glass of water or fresh orange juice instead. If possible, take a walk or jog around outside in the fresh air for a few minutes. At

the very least, have a good stretch – this gets the oxygen circulating around your body, gives you fresh energy and stops rising panic.

2 Vent your spleen. If it's feasible, shouting, screaming or groaning is a marvellous way of releasing stress. If you can't do it literally, pretend you're doing it – we hold a lot of tension in our jaws and the action of screaming or groaning is a great way to release that tension. Invest in a punchbag for the home or workplace, wherever, and give it a good thump or six. Exercise classes such as Boxercise and Tai-Bo can be brilliant ways of alleviating stress. So, too, can all the martial arts.

3 Practise constructive vandalism: beat the hell out of bubblewrap. It sounds acutely weird, but studies have shown that popping bubblewrap (apparently, the big bubbles work best) dispels pent-up nervous energy and muscle tension.

Strategies for medium-term stress

If you regularly find yourself at boiling point, it's time to adopt some longer-term self-preservation techniques.

1 Adopt a good-mood diet. Doctors have always recommended regular meals to combat stress, but now they know that the foods we eat can truly affect our mental state. Depression, anxiety, an inability to concentrate, panic attacks, mood swings, forgetfulness and lethargy – all symptoms of stress – can be triggered by sensitivity to certain foods. The anti-stress diet is high in fruit, vegetables, legumes, nuts and grains. In particular, grapes, millet, wheat germ, brewer's yeast, oats, molasses and buckwheat are touted as anti-stress superfoods. Foods to avoid include all refined carbohydrates, sugar, tea and coffee, sweetened commercial drinks and excess bran.

2 Exercise – strenuously. A good, tough aerobic workout can release stress like virtually nothing else. When the body cannot rid itself of the excess hormones generated by stress, the result is a harmful state in which the mind and body are permanently aroused. If you're stuck in this twilight zone, you need to kick yourself into a state of pure physical, rather than pure mental, arousal. You can then swing back into the state we know as rest.

3 Float. Regularly floating in the equivalent of an isolation tank is one of the best stress-busters going. Not only does it relieve stress, but it also enhances creativity, decision making and problem solving (see pages 11–12).

4 Have sex! Seriously. Researchers think that orgasm may be a release mechanism for the body, in a similar manner to other body reactions such as laughing and crying. It appears that sex defuses the chemicals produced by stress in much the same way as intense exercise. During lovemaking, the muscles of the body become highly tensed; after orgasm, the body completely relaxes: it's like a very extreme version of the relaxation exercise known as progressive relaxation, where you move through the body tensing and then relaxing each set of muscles. During sex, your body does this automatically and to a much greater degree. More information on good sex is given Chapter 8.

Long-term solutions for deep, dark stress

1 Delegate. You're not superman or superwoman – you cannot do absolutely everything and, believe it or not, the world will not fall apart if you say no occasionally. Stress-management counsellors all recommend taking stock of your life and deciding what's important and what can go by the wayside. Write a list of what causes you stress and consider if there is anything that you can drop or delegate.

2 Meditate or practise mindfulness (see pages 14–16). Try these techniques if you feel stress taking over your life.

3 Practise mental circuit training. If meditation seems too far-out and mystical, follow the example of cosmonauts and astronauts, airline pilots and Olympic athletes: learn autogenic training. Autogenic training is recognized as one of the finest stress-busters in the Western world. It gives you instant stress relief wherever and whenever you need it, lowers blood pressure and cholesterol, relieves insomnia and eases migraine. Yet it is easy to learn and, afterwards, you need only spend a few minutes a day on the exercises – or use them when you feel yourself becoming severely stressed. See pages 16–18.

4 Factor in 'time out' during each and every day. It need only be 5 minutes in the morning and afternoon, but stick to this religiously. Use it to lie down and relax, or place your palms over your eyes and lean forwards on your desk. Even short pauses can break the stress pattern.

If, after trying these strategies, you still find stress is ruling your life, seek expert help. Try your doctor first – he or she may be able to refer you to a psychologist specializing in stress management. Otherwise, the psychological associations or your natural health centre should be able to put you in touch with someone who can help.

Be kind to yourself

Pampering yourself is a brilliant way to beat stress. Think about the following.

1 Set aside a small amount of time every day to do something just for you. It could be an hour's massage; half an hour soaking in the bath with soft music, candles and exotic oils; or simply quarter of an hour curled up in a chair with a novel or a magazine.

2 Make a list of the ten things that give you the most pleasure and embed them in your life on a regular basis.

3 Take frequent open-air breaks. Borrow a dog for a walk in the park; meet friends for a picnic or hike, rather than lunch or the cinema.

4 Surround yourself with people who support you. Often we see people because we feel obliged to or so we don't hurt their feelings. Think honestly about your friends – about who makes you feel relaxed and good about yourself. Choose whom you really want to see.

5 Place yourself in a calm, nourishing environment. Whether you live in a big house or one small room, make it your personal haven. A lit candle lifts a room's energy and is calming and soothing. Treat yourself to fresh flowers.

6 Acknowledge the stress in your life but don't let it rule you. Be gentle on yourself and approve of yourself – it's incredible how much stress we create for ourselves by disliking ourselves and giving ourselves a hard time.

7 Smile. Smiling automatically releases endorphins, chemical feelgood messages to the brain, so you almost instantly feel less stressed.

Floating

Lying in pitch darkness and utter silence in 45 cm (18 in) of highly salted water sounds a strange way to beat stress. Yet floating is one of the very best (and certainly one of the most pleasant) ways of stressbusting.

The principle behind floating is simple. It was developed in the 1950s by Dr John C. Lilly, a medical doctor who was also trained as a psychoanalyst and a specialist in neurophysiology. Lilly was intrigued by what happened to the brain and body when all external stimuli were removed, and conducted experiments in the soundproof chambers that the navy used to train its divers. From this, he developed his own tank and continued his research. The results were far-reaching – many said far-fetched. People who floated claimed they thought and worked better, could learn more easily and concentrate better. Some said their creativity improved; others even said they felt younger and healthier. Some claimed their sex lives rocketed. Almost without exception, participants insisted they felt much more calm and relaxed.

Several centres in the USA have spent the past 20 years analysing what actually happens when we float. Their results have shown that floating can indeed do all those things – and more. The almost complete sensory deprivation caused by floating seems to agree with both our bodies and our minds.

What can floating help?

- Blood pressure and heart rate fall, while oxygen consumption improves.
- People suffering chronic pain find that they can obtain relief, often not just for the time they float, but for up to 3 days afterwards. Research suggests this can be attributed to the way floating stimulates the body to produce endorphins, natural painkillers.
- Musicians, actors and writers frequently float because floating allows the right hemisphere of the brain to operate freely, leading to much more creativity and imagination, and improving the ability to solve problems.
- Students revising for exams float while listening to tapes of their revision material – the 'superlearning' effect of floating helps them take in far more than a normal hour's study.
- Many psychotherapists find that therapy is much more effective with the client in a tank, rather than on the couch: not only do clients relax quickly, but also they find it much easier to recall past experiences and are much more responsive to positive suggestions and visualizations.
- One of floating's most successful applications is in the treatment of addictive behaviour: overeating, smoking, drug taking and alcoholism all respond remarkably well.
- Phobias often clear up quickly and anxiety states frequently disappear altogether.

What can I expect from a session?

WHERE WILL I HAVE THE TREATMENT?
You will be lying in around 45 cm (18 in) of highly salted warm water in a darkened cubicle. These cubicles range in size, although most are small.

WILL I BE CLOTHED?
You will be either naked or wearing a swimming costume.

WHAT HAPPENS?

The procedure will be explained to you and then usually you will be left by yourself. You get undressed, shower and step into the tank. You then lie with your head propped on an inflatable pillow. Some centres will play music (or you can bring your own tapes) or you can float in silence. There will be a prearranged signal when your time is coming to an end. After this, you simply get out, shower again and get dressed. Usually, you will relax for at least a short time to allow yourself to 'come to'.

WILL IT HURT?

No, it does not hurt at all. It's actually very pleasant.

WILL ANYTHING STRANGE HAPPEN?

You may spontaneously recall childhood incidents or suddenly find solutions to tricky problems. Some people report almost 'out-of-body' experiences. You may fall asleep and dream vividly.

Do-it-yourself flotation

Flotation tanks are expensive – and do take up room. If you don't have your own or can't get to a flotation centre, you can still enjoy the healing and relaxing effects of Epsom salts.

1 Dissolve about 450 g (1 lb) of Epsom salts in a warm bath, then allow yourself to soak.
2 Relax for about 20 minutes. Drink a hot herbal tea (thyme or peppermint would be ideal) while soaking, to increase perspiration and replace lost fluids.
3 Be extra careful as you get out of the bath – you may feel light-headed.
4 Do not rub yourself dry. Wrap up in several large towels and go to bed, making sure you wrap your feet warmly.
5 In the morning, or when you wake, sponge yourself down with warm water. Rub your body vigorously dry.

CAUTION: avoid Epsom salts baths if you have heart trouble, if you are diabetic or if you are feeling tired or weak.

2 Meditation

Meditation, the art of stilling the mind, has been practised for literally thousands of years. It is a remarkably straightforward technique which can fit into our daily lives with the greatest of ease. In recent years, meditation has been scientifically recognized as being highly effective in treating a range of problems, both physiological and psychological.

From the Indian tradition of yoga to orthodox Christianity, from the mountains of Tibet to the plains of the USA, various forms of meditation have been used for millennia. It began as a religious practice, similar to contemplative prayer, but, over the centuries, it became obvious that meditation's benefits stretch way beyond the spiritual.

Meditation is simply a means of creating calm in the mind. Stop for a moment and become aware of your thoughts. They will probably be jumping all over the place; odd worries, concerns and images will spring into your mind. Meditation, however, helps us train the mind to filter out the unwanted chatter of everyday life, taking us to a still, peaceful place where both mind and body can fully relax. Many meditators find that just 20 minutes of meditation is as refreshing as several hours' sleep. This happens because the deep relaxation that meditation brings about puts our brains into a particularly restful frequency, akin to deep sleep.

The ancient yogis said that meditation was a powerful tonic which produced an acceleration of energy in the body, rejuvenating cells and holding back the ravages of time. For thousands of years, disciples had to take their word for it, but now science is proving that meditation really is potent medicine. Hundreds of scientific studies into meditation have produced impressive evidence. Researchers have found that meditation reduces hypertension, serum cholesterol and blood cortisol, which is related to stress in the body. It has been found effective in reducing the effects of angina, allergies, chronic headaches, diabetes and bronchial asthma, and can help lessen dependence on alcohol and cigarettes. Meditators, researchers found, see their doctors less and spend 70 per cent fewer days in hospital. Anxiety, depression and irritability all decrease, while memory improves and reaction times become faster. Meditation, it appears, gives us more stamina, a happier disposition and even helps us enjoy better relationships.

How to meditate

Meditation is simplicity itself to practise. An experienced meditator can meditate anytime, anywhere. When you first start to meditate, however, it can be very helpful to choose a place that is quiet and warm, one where you will not be disturbed. Ideally, you should be seated – in whatever position you find comfortable. That might be on the floor, cross-legged, perhaps sitting on a cushion. It could equally be sitting upright in a supportive chair with your hands resting gently on your knees. It's not a good idea to meditate lying down, as you may well fall asleep.

You don't actually need any props at all for meditation, although some people find it helps to watch the flickering flame of a candle. However, for most meditation, it is usual to keep your eyes gently shut to cut out external stimuli.

The easiest way to start meditating is to join a class. There are all kinds of meditation, to suit every disposition. Many yoga classes incorporate meditation using sound or breathing to focus the mind. There are classes available in chanting – from Eastern mantras to over-tone chanting (as in Gregorian chant). Some classes advocate meditating on a word or symbol reflecting your personal spiritual beliefs. But you can learn to meditate on your own if you prefer. All it takes is a quiet room, 20 minutes and a touch of self-discipline.

Basic meditation exercise

1 Sit with an alert yet relaxed body posture, making sure you feel comfortable (either in a straight-backed chair with your feet flat on the floor or on a thick, firm cushion, 7.5–15 cm (3–6 in) off the floor).
2 Keep your back straight, aligned with your head and neck, and relax your body.
3 Start to breathe steadily and deeply. Notice your breathing and observe the breath as it flows in and out, feeling your abdomen falling and rising. Give it your full attention.
4 If you find your attention starts to wander, simply note the fact and gently bring your thoughts back to your breathing, to the rising and falling of your abdomen.
5 Always try to sit for around 20 minutes. Don't jump up immediately afterwards. Bring yourself back to normal consciousness slowly. Become aware of the room around you, gently stretch and 'come back' fully before standing up.

There are many different ways of meditating. If the exercise above does not suit you, you could try these alternatives:

• **CANDLE MEDITATION** Sit in front of a lit candle. Focus your eyes on the flame and watch it. Keep your attention on the flame.

• **COUNTING MEDITATION** Slowly count from one to ten in your head, keeping your attention on each number. If you feel your attention wandering (undoubtedly it will!), simply go back to one and start again.

• **SOUND MEDITATION** Choose a sacred sound, a favourite word or phrase. It could be something like 'ohm' or 'shalom', a vowel sound like 'aaaah' or a phrase such as 'I am at peace' or 'The Lord is my Shepherd'. Choose one that has meaning for you. Quietly repeat it – experiment to find the best way.

NOTE: most people should have absolutely no problems meditating, but it is worth mentioning that, in isolated cases, people have experienced negative effects. The act of still-ing the mind can sometimes bring repressed memories to the surface. These can prove disturbing; if this occurs, consult a trained counsellor or psychotherapist. There have been very rare instances of people suffering quite severe psychological disturbances. These seem confined, however, to people who have a history of psychological illness.

Mindfulness

We spend our lives trying to be happy, but often end up chasing our own tails. We project happiness into the future, promising ourselves that we would be happy if only we could win the lottery, get a better job, a nicer house, less stress, more money ... Yet the key to true happiness lies not in the outside world, but deep within. Mindfulness is meditation brought up to date, pared of its mystical and religious connotations and honed to slot into the most frenetic Western lifestyle. The simple idea is to give people control of their lives by teaching them how to listen to their minds and bodies, rather than be tossed around by the world outside.

Mindfulness is the brainwave of Jon Kabat-Zinn, the scientist with a PhD in molecular biology who runs the Stress Reduction Clinic at the University of Massachusetts Hospital. The clinic was started in 1979 in the light of a realization that, although the hospital could treat patients with chronic physical ailments, their problems would recur after a while. Kabat-Zinn felt sure that the answer lay in teaching patients how to kickstart their own healing powers. He spent years finding the best and most straightforward method. His choice lay in Buddhist and yogic practices, which he then adapted for Western consumption. The results have been impressive: he has found his form of meditation can help to clear psoriasis much faster, can relieve chronic pain and can also lessen feelings of anxiety and depression. He has instructed patients whose illnesses range from heart disease to ulcerative colitis, from diabetes to cancer. 'We teach these people to develop an intimacy and familiarity with their own bodies and minds,' he explains. 'This leads to a greater confidence to learn from their symptoms and to begin to self-regulate them.'

You don't need to be sick to benefit from mindfulness meditation. Its simple techniques can help everyone live life with greater certainty and self-confidence. At its most basic level, mindfulness simply involves stopping and becoming aware of the moment. The easiest way to do this is to focus on your breathing, gently letting go any stray thoughts or worries that emerge. Kabat-Zinn asks his patients to strive for 45 minutes of mindfulness a day, but stresses that even a few minutes makes a great difference. 'It can be 5 minutes or even 5 seconds,' he says, 'but for those moments, don't try to change anything at all, just breathe and let go. Give yourself permission to allow this moment to be exactly as it is and allow yourself to be exactly as you are.'

Mindfulness may be simple, but it is not necessarily easy, he warns. Not only does it require effort and discipline, but also the very act of stopping and listening can often summon up deep emotions such as grief, sadness, anger and fear that have been unconsciously suppressed over the years. Equally, however, it can summon up feelings such as joy, peacefulness and happiness. Many people find that it helps them to discover what they really want from life.

Making mindfulness work for you

- Make mindfulness the very first thing you do each day. Wake up a little earlier than usual and, before you even move, notice your breathing; breathe consciously for a few minutes. Feel your body lying in bed and then straighten it out and stretch. Try to think of the day ahead as an adventure, filled with possibilities. Remember, you can never really foresee what the day will hold.
- Try stopping, sitting down and becoming aware of your breathing once in a while throughout the day. It can be for 5 minutes or even 5 seconds. Just breathe and let go – allow yourself to be exactly as you are.
- Set aside a time every day to just be: 5 minutes would be fine, or 20 or 30. Sit and become aware of your breathing; every time your mind wanders, simply return to the breath.
- Use your mindfulness time to contemplate what you really want from life. Ask yourself questions: 'Who am I?', 'Where am I going?', 'If I could choose a path now, in

which direction would I head?' or 'What do I truly love?' You don't have to come up with answers, just persist with the asking.

- Try getting down on the floor once a day and stretching your body mindfully, if only for a few minutes. Stay in touch with your breathing and listen to what your body has to tell you.
- Use ordinary occasions to become mindful. When you are in the shower, really feel the water on the skin, rather than losing yourself in thought. When you eat, really taste your food. Notice how you feel when the telephone rings.
- Practise kindness to yourself. As you sit and breathe, invite a sense of self-acceptance and cherishing to arise in your heart. If it starts to go away, gently bring it back. Imagine you are being held in the arms of a loving parent, completely accepted and completely loved.

Autogenic training

Autogenic training (AT) has been dubbed 'meditation for Westerners'. It consists of a series of simple mental exercises designed to switch off the 'fight or flight' stress mechanism of the body and allow you to deal with the traumas of the day coolly, calmly and in total control. It's the ideal choice for anyone who wants a scientifically researched, simple and straightforward, streamlined method of stress relief.

Autogenic training originated in Germany in the 1920s and was formulated by a Berlin doctor, Dr Johannes Schultz. Another German, Dr Wolfgang Luthe, took the concept of autogenic training and developed it into its current form. More than 3,000 scientific publications have run reports on the beneficial effects of autogenic training, making it one of the best-documented and most consistently researched methods of stress relief in the world.

So what does this mind workout comprise? Quite simply, it's a case of learning how to focus your attention inwards through a series of mental exercises. There are three basic components: first, the art of passive concentration (quietly allowing your mind to focus on your body); secondly, the repetition of certain phrases or words that allow you to target certain parts of the body and induce feelings such as heaviness or warmth; and, thirdly, the positioning of your body into certain standard postures to cut out the effects of the outside world. The three positions involve lying flat on the floor in a totally relaxed position (somewhat akin to a yoga asana); sitting in a chair with your hands resting on the arms of the chair or on your thighs; or perching on the edge of a hard chair in a kind of slump, with the back and head loosely drooping forwards.

It's a highly flexible system: once you've learnt it, you can practise it sitting in your office, on the train, in a parked car or lying in bed. Next, you are taught how to focus on sensations in the body, imagining warmth in the arms and legs. Breathing is calm and easy; you learn how just to watch your breathing, rather than trying to control it. Simply thinking about the exercises makes you feel calm.

The system is taught in weekly one-hour sessions over a period of 8 weeks. People generally find they become far calmer, easier and more relaxed. They sleep better, too.

Sportspeople have found that their performance improves with autogenic training. Creativity seems to shoot up and many businesspeople discover that not only do their stress levels drop, but also their communication skills and ability to make clear, effective decisions improve dramatically. The reason, apparently, is that autogenic training brings the two sides of the brain into better balance, allowing you the benefit of the intuitive, imaginative right side of the brain, which is normally switched firmly off during waking life.

In addition, when you practise autogenic training, you tend to need, on average, an hour's less sleep at night.

You should always be taught this technique by a fully qualified teacher. Not only should everyone have a medical consultation before starting the course, but also it has to be emphasized that this is not a superficial cosmetic relaxation technique: it works at a very deep level. Aside from the sheer physical effects that autogenic training can have, it can also work profoundly on the mind. Sometimes, hitherto deep-hidden anxieties, feelings of anger or frustration can surface when you start the training. Occasionally, people report headaches or chest pains. It is clearly very important to have qualified advice on hand.

What can autogenic training help?

- People report feeling calmer and more able to cope through the use of autogenic training; they are in control of their lives, rather than feeling that life is controlling them.
- Autogenic training has been proven to relieve tension and insomnia significantly and to lessen anxiety.
- It lowers both blood pressure and blood cholesterol (a key measure in preventing heart attacks). In fact, its effects can be so dramatic that people with medical conditions have to be carefully monitored while they train. Some diabetics have found they needed to halve the amount of insulin they take when they practise autogenic training, and other forms of medication can also be decreased in dosage in many cases.
- It is helpful in psychosomatic disorders and has been used to help people with cancer.
- There has been early work with infertility – it was found that a significant number of women have high levels of the stress hormone prolactin, which acts as a natural contraceptive and stops conception. When they practised autogenic training, these women found the hormone levels dropped and a good proportion conceived. The benefits continue after conception: pregnant women who practise autogenic training report that it reduces the stress of childbirth.
- Many airlines use the technique to combat insomnia and jetlag in their staff, and it is used quite widely in other industries to reduce stress and improve performance at all levels. Autogenic training has even been taught to astronauts and cosmonauts, as part of their space-training programmes.
- Some therapists are experimenting with using it to counter the effects of Parkinson's disease.

What can I expect from a session?

WHERE WILL I HAVE THE TREATMENT?
You will be sitting on an upright chair, relaxed in an easy chair or lying on a couch or the floor (the three ways of practising autogenic training).

WILL I BE CLOTHED?
Yes, you remain fully clothed throughout.

WHAT HAPPENS?
The teacher will explain clearly how autogenic training works. Each week, you will focus on a different part of the body and learn how to get in touch with it and how to gain an element of control over its degree of relaxation. For example, to begin with, you will work at inducing a feeling of heaviness and relaxation in your arms, later learning to spread this feeling to

all your limbs. You will then learn to regulate your heartbeat and breathing, bring softness to the solar plexus, relax tension in your shoulders and feel coolness on your brow.

As the weeks progress, you will learn how to combine the various commands into a system of inducing complete relaxation throughout your whole body and mind.

WILL IT HURT?
No, there is nothing painful about autogenic training.

WILL ANYTHING STRANGE HAPPEN?
Some people feel slightly uncomfortable about getting in touch with their heartbeat or breathing. You may find the process stirs up old emotions.

WILL I BE GIVEN ANYTHING TO TAKE?
No, medication is not a part of the treatment.

IS THERE ANY HOMEWORK?
Yes, between lessons, you will be expected to practise autogenic training exercises several times during the day. The more you practise, the more effective the treatment.

Do-it-yourself autogenic training

To get the most from autogenic training, you need to be taught the technique individually. However, these relaxation tips are based on its philosophy.

1 Sit down and close your eyes for a moment. Practise quiet observation of yourself. Check for body tension: are you clenching any muscles? Don't try to change anything; just be aware of it. If you have an ache or pain, such as a headache, quietly observe it. Decide that it is a form of stress release that may be beneficial. Rather than seeing it as a problem, take an interest in its movements or intensity. Watch your breathing. Let it lead you wherever it wants, whether in the form of sighs, shallow panting or quiet abdominal breathing. Don't change it; just go along with it.

2 When you feel tense or upset, retreat to somewhere private, such as your bedroom or bathroom, and 'shake' it out of your system. Loosely shake each limb in turn and feel the wobble. When you catch yourself saying 'I could scream', do it. Bury your face in a pillow and let rip. No one will hear you and you'll feel much better. If you need to cry and can't, make some moaning sounds with dry sobs and you may start yourself off. Think how a child cries automatically – at times we need to relearn natural responses.

3 Have some fun. When did you last have a really good laugh? Ring up a friend and arrange a crazy night out. Go to a show: let some playtime back in your life. Above all, allow yourself to believe you're a worthwhile person, warts and all. Decide that your feelings are part of you. Express them safely and honestly (in private), then turn your thoughts to a more positive outlook.

4 Quietly become aware of your heartbeat. Don't try to alter anything: just be aware. Think of what an amazing job your heart does. You can continue this awareness by focusing on your breathing. Notice how you breathe. How far do you take the air into your lungs? Do you breathe deeply or shallowly? Make sure you take this exercise very slowly and carefully – if you feel uncomfortable at any point, stop.

3 Talking Therapies

Not long ago, no one would ever admit to seeing a psychotherapist or psychiatrist – it was tantamount to admitting you were insane. Now the situation is different. Psychotherapy has become acceptable – in some places, even fashionable. But do you really need it? In the past, you would see a mind therapist only if you had severe depression or mania, or a phobia that prevented you from getting on with your life. Nowadays, people see therapists for a host of reasons – some serious, some seemingly quite trivial.

The whole issue of psychotherapy is complex. Many seemingly psychological problems disappear when you adjust your diet and start to exercise. Lots of people have found they have been 'cured' of their depression with a simple prescription of regular exercise. Equally, many others have found 'mental' problems such as anxiety or irritability miraculously disappear when they shift to a healthy wholefood diet. Shyness, lack of confidence and poor self-esteem can gradually dissipate when people start an exercise programme.

When problems seem intractable, however, you may decide that some form of psychotherapy could help you clarify your life and sort out the problems. If this is the case, trust your instincts and find yourself a therapist. Do bear in mind that psychotherapists aren't gods – they can't wave a magic wand and sort out your problems for you. They are not there to give you the answers on a plate, but to help you find the answers for yourself.

There are as many different forms of psychotherapy as there are days in the year and the mere idea of choosing a therapist can be as off-putting as ordering from a very long menu in a completely foreign language. Should you go for psychodrama or psychosynthesis? What is the difference between primal integration and primal therapy, or even primal integration and postural integration? Psychobabble? It's a veritable Tower of Babel.

All therapies do, however, have one basic aim: to make you feel better about yourself, to help you get the most out of life. It is just that they approach it in very different ways.

The four major approaches

Let's try to clarify what's on offer. As far as psychotherapy proper goes, there are basically four main approaches: psychoanalytic, behavioural, cognitive and humanistic.

- **Psychoanalysis** follows the patterns laid down by Sigmund Freud. He believed that our behaviour is influenced as much by the unconscious as the conscious mind and that certain instinctual urges, such as aggression or sex, are often driven into the unconscious.
- **Behavioural psychotherapy** teaches that the environment 'conditions' people to behave in certain ways and that we all adapt our responses to fit in with our surroundings. In other words, if you reward someone for doing well, they will continue to do well; if you reward them when they fail, they will continue to fail.

- **Cognitive psychotherapy** contends that we make sense of our world via specific views and assumptions that have been learnt, or conditioned, by our earlier experiences. By changing our beliefs and attitudes, it teaches, we can change our behaviour.
- **Humanistic psychology** is the umbrella name for a collection of approaches tied together by shared beliefs. Emphasis is put on how we as individuals experience the world and the sense we make of it, with particular regard to self-esteem, self-awareness and feelings. Generally included are the existential approaches, the work of Abraham Maslow, Thomas Szasz and Ronald Laing. It is also bound up with the human potential movement and encounter.

Most therapists will practise one of these four approaches or a combination. However, there are literally hundreds of offshoots and subschools, all with their own theories. Also, don't forget that bodywork therapies (see *Therapies for a Healthy Body*, another title in this series) can have a psychotherapeutic effect, as can many of the more creative therapies that are investigated later on in this section. To make things more complicated, no two therapists will work in exactly the same way, even when ostensibly practising the same therapy.

How should you choose your therapy?

It may sound unscientific, but really the only way is to read about the different approaches to see which, if any, appeal. Next, send off for their literature to get more precise, detailed information. Many centres organize introductory events such as lectures or workshops. If you prefer the idea of one-to-one therapy, good therapists should be only too happy to give an introductory session to see if you get on with one another. Umbrella organizations such as those listed at the back of the book can also offer advice.

How much you can afford is another pertinent question. Traditional one-to-one analysis and psychotherapy demand a long-term cash commitment. Group work is cheaper and often runs in courses. Some approaches consist of a set number of sessions, so the expenditure has an end in sight. At the other end of the scale, co-counselling costs virtually nothing once you are trained.

Often there's a temptation to decide on the kind of therapy that matches your personality. Precise, strait-laced people tend to be drawn to the rigour and order of analysis; creative, expressive people may well feel happier with a more expansive therapy such as dance or primal therapy. Yet people who intellectualize too much may well derive numerous benefits from a 'non-intellectual' approach such as dance, while the expressive types may find a more logical approach interesting and challenging.

Ask yourself in what kind of situation you would feel most comfortable. Many people find the idea of talking about their feelings in a group terrifying; for others, there is 'safety in numbers'. Some like the idea of hitting emotions head-on in confrontational therapies such as encounter or primal. Introverted people who are scared of expressing themselves may find a gentle approach such as art just what they need.

The major decision you face is group versus individual therapy. One-to-one therapy is a natural choice if you find the idea of groups frightening or have difficulty forming close relationships: ideally, you will develop a bond with your therapist and you will be able to discuss personal matters in confidence. Group therapy also has advantages. It provides feedback from varying types of people, not just the therapist. It also enables the therapist to observe you in a more natural situation, interacting with the other members of the group. Equally importantly, it gives you a chance to see that you're not alone in your problems: realizing that other people have equally difficult lives can make you feel far less isolated.

Most people still opt for a 'talking' therapy – analysis, psychotherapy etc. – but this is by no means the only option. You can also choose therapies that don't demand you probe your psyche directly. For example, in creative therapies such as dance, you do not have to talk at great length about yourself.

There is a theory that, as long as you really want it to work, virtually any therapy will do the trick. It really is a case of finding an approach that interests you and that you feel would be of the most benefit to you. Some would say that you will be subconsciously drawn to the right one!

A brief A–Z of therapies

This is a necessarily short introductory outline of the major types of therapy you are likely to come across.

ADLERIAN PSYCHOLOGY (INDIVIDUAL PSYCHOLOGY): Adlerian counsellors see each person as driven by his or her self-chosen goals – often based on how we perceived life as children. Adler saw life as having three main tasks: work, relationships and society/the community. The therapy is carried out either one-to-one or in groups or workshops.

ART THERAPY: See pages 65–6.

ASTROLOGICAL COUNSELLING: Carl Jung began the interest in astrology as part of psychological healing; now there is a growing trend towards combining astrology and counselling. Basically, this holds that the planets' positions can influence the client's personality and life. Through counselling and interpretation of the client's birth chart, insights are given and advice offered. Sometimes the counsellor will draw up charts for partners or other significant people in the client's life to see where conflicts and problems occur.

BIOENERGETICS OR BIOENERGETIC THERAPY: This is a body-orientated form of therapy based on the belief that the body, mind and emotions are linked – by observing tensions in the body, you can diagnose problems within the psyche. Releasing these bodily tensions means emotional issues will surface to be resolved. Therapy involves exercises to release tense muscles; great attention is given to breathing, movement and voicing. Bioenergetics can be learnt in groups or one-to-one.

CLIENT-CENTRED THERAPY: Developed by Carl Rogers, this is sometimes known as Rogerian counselling. Practised either one-to-one or in groups, it has at its core a belief that the client's view of the world is always valid: the therapist will not try to interpret the clients' behaviour or change the way they see themselves. This is a gentle therapy in which the therapist listens with empathy to the client and then seeks to reflect the thoughts and feelings expressed.

CO-COUNSELLING: This is a form of do-it-yourself counselling in which two non-professionals counsel one another. One takes on the role of client; the other becomes the therapist. After an agreed length of time, they switch places. Training courses in co-counselling last about 40 hours. You can then join a network which puts you in touch with prospective partners.

COUNSELLING: This term is widely used for a huge variety of approaches. Counselling can simply involve quiet listening, advice-giving or comforting, or it may mean psychotherapy.

COUPLE THERAPY: Offered to all couples, regardless of marital status or sexual orientation, couple therapy attempts to resolve conflict within a relationship. Both partners are required to attend so that both sides of the problem can be observed. Many people find it a very useful way to talk about their feelings and hurts without the process degenerating into argument. If there are children, they are often involved, too.

DANCE THERAPY: See pages 61–2.

DRAMA THERAPY: Often used for the physically and mentally challenged and for children with severe behavioural problems, drama therapy is another of the creative therapies that offers a safe environment for exploring potentially difficult emotions.

DREAM THERAPY: See Chapter 10.

EYE MOVEMENT DESENSITIZATION AND REPROCESSING (EMDR): This relatively new therapy from the USA appears to be having swift and profound effects in treating phobias and post-traumatic stress. The therapist flicks a finger back and forth in front of the patient's eyes; the patient follows the movement and brings to mind what is causing the problem.

EXISTENTIAL PSYCHOTHERAPY: Quite unlike most other psychotherapies, this is as much about digesting existential philosophy as it is about coming to terms with oneself. Existentialism looks at the 'big' questions of life: death, alienation, suffering, responsibility. Not an easy approach, it appeals to those interested in the philosophy and writings of Friedrich Nietzsche, Jean-Paul Sartre, Martin Heidegger et al.

FAMILY THERAPY: Often used when a child in a family has problems, the therapy focuses not on the individual, but the family as a whole. The entire family is included in therapy and one or two therapists assist. It is mostly carried out within child guidance units, psychiatric departments and social services.

FLOWER REMEDY THERAPY: Highly diluted essences of flowers are believed to influence your mood and emotional state. Therapists will ask questions to determine the client's predominant state and then prescribe different essences. Flower remedies are usually used with other forms of therapy – frequently counselling or hypnosis. See pages 69–71.

GESTALT: Dissatisfied with Freudian psychoanalysis, Fritz and Laura Perls evolved Gestalt therapy in the 1960s. The focus shifted from the verbal to the non-verbal, with more attention being paid to how people behave than what they say. Gestalt therapy is usually conducted in groups.

GROUP-ORIENTATED PSYCHOTHERAPY: This umbrella term covers therapy in which working within a group framework is considered useful and therapeutic. Rather than being simply therapy carried out in a group, the group becomes a key part of the therapy. Often the therapist stays in the background. The group may simply free-associate or members may focus on what is happening in their lives at that moment.

HYPNOTHERAPY: This involves the therapist leading the client into a state of deep relaxation. From here, the therapist may simply offer positive statements to the subconscious mind or involve the client in a more dynamic experience, exploring feelings, re-enacting situations or going back into dreams to discover their messages. The client is always aware of what is going on and never loses control.

JUNGIAN PSYCHOTHERAPY (ANALYSIS): Carl Jung widened Freud's idea of the unconscious, believing that, apart from the individual unconscious, we all share a 'collective unconscious', a vast pool of shared knowledge and feelings. Jung believed we need to integrate our conscious and unconscious minds, and worked with dreams, fantasies and symbols. Central themes include the exploration of archetypes (the shadow, the wise person etc.); the relationship between our masculine and feminine sides (the animus and anima); and the power of myth. Jungian analysis is conducted one-to-one, with the analyst and client sitting upright facing each other. There is less focus on the past, more on the present and future.

KLEINIAN PSYCHOTHERAPY (ANALYSIS): Following the work of Freud, Melanie Klein focused on the importance of the early years of life. Her central theory was that, as babies, we feel conflicting emotions of love and hate, primarily towards our mothers. These conflicts remain unresolved and create tension in later life. Kleinian analysts encourage clients to express good *and* bad feelings, transferring them from the mother to the analyst, so that they can be explored and understood.

MEN'S THERAPY: A response to women's therapy, men's groups have suffered a certain amount of ridicule (with images of naked men beating their chests and banging drums in the woods). However, the rationale is as valid as that for all-women groups: sometimes it can be much easier to discuss painful issues within same-sex groups. Men's therapy is always conducted in groups, although each group may have a different emphasis. Some focus specifically on the issue of masculinity, while others discuss more general concerns.

MUSIC THERAPY: Music can easily change or affect mood and so has wide applications in therapy. It is often used to release feelings and to help those with physical or mental disabilities.

NEURO-LINGUISTIC PROGRAMMING (NLP): See pages 29–31.

OPEN ENCOUNTER (ENCOUNTER): This group therapy encourages people to forget about what is and isn't 'done' in 'polite society' and to explore their true feelings. It has no rigid format: the group will deal with whatever emotions or impulses arise. Sometimes this involves truthful speaking; at others, physical activity such as kicking or beating a cushion.

PERSONAL CONSTRUCT THERAPY: This therapy has some novel attributes. It usually starts with self-characterization – the client writing a biography of himself or herself as if it had been written by a good friend. From this, the analyst evaluates the client's self-image then creates a fictional character who views the world in a totally different way from the client. The client is then asked to 'be' this character for a week.

PRIMAL INTEGRATION: This is a quite separate entity from primal therapy. Practitioners do not see it as a therapy as such, but rather as a growth process, a journey of self-development which incorporates elements of a spiritual path. Like most forms of therapy, the aim is integration, becoming whole. Practitioners use a variety of methods, including physical therapies and investigating feelings, dreams and fantasies.

PRIMAL THERAPY: Arthur Janov held that unhappiness and neurosis are caused by deep-seated childhood pain. Primal therapists believe that this can be exorcised by reliving it. The focus is on the client's hurt and any incidents of abuse or neglect. Clients are encouraged to release their pain in any way they like – curling up and crying, or screaming and punching cushions. The therapist acts as support. It is quite intense: for 3 weeks, the client is seen every day for up to 3 hours. A more relaxed programme is then followed for a year.

PSYCHOANALYSIS: Founded by Sigmund Freud, this is the archetypal image of therapy à la Woody Allen: the highly charged relationship with the 'shrink', the couch, the transference of emotions connected with figures from your life on to the analyst, the concept of resistance (withholding key feelings). Very formal and highly structured, it requires a huge investment of time, effort and money. The analyst and or patient sees the analyst four or five times a week for several years. The patient lies on a couch, with the analyst sitting behind or out of direct eye contact, and is asked simply to talk or free-associate, saying whatever comes to mind.

PSYCHOANALYTIC PSYCHOTHERAPY: This is a watered-down, more practical version of full-scale analysis which still follows Freud's principles. Sessions tend to be once or twice a week and the patient and analyst generally sit facing each other.

PSYCHODRAMA: If you feel as if you live life like an actor on a stage, psychodrama may well appeal. Its creator, Jacob Moreno, felt that 'all the world's a stage'; psychodrama is group psychotherapy combined with theatre. The 'director' (therapist) encourages the 'protagonist' to re-enact scenes from his or her life, while other members of the group take on the supporting roles. Ideally, fresh insights will occur and a form of catharsis follows.

PSYCHOSYNTHESIS: Roberto Assagioli trained in Freudian analysis, but focused on the 'higher' unconscious – the source of inspiration, joy and peak experiences. He sought to blend the concepts of Western psychology and Eastern mysticism. Psychosynthesis aims to draw together all the different roles we play, all the warring, contradictory parts of the psyche. A variety of techniques is used, from painting and drawing to guided imagery and engaging in inner dialogues with different parts of your self.

SOLUTION THERAPY (SOLUTION-FOCUSED OR BRIEF THERAPY): See page 27–9.

TRANSACTIONAL ANALYSIS: A Canadian psychotherapist, Eric Berne, developed transactional analysis and, in 1964, wrote the bestselling book *Games People Play*. His theory is that we live our lives according to scripts that originate in childhood, but which affect our whole lives. Examples would be 'Be Perfect', in which we always feel we should do better, or 'Hurry Up', where we always feel we are running out of time. By learning to identify and understand our hardwired scripts, we can understand and change our behaviour. Initial sessions involve learning the theory and the language of transactional analysis. It is usually conducted in groups.

TRANSPERSONAL PSYCHOTHERAPY: This is a branch of psychotherapy that emphasizes the spiritual and the search for meaning in life. The key concept is the idea of self or the soul, which seeks to unite itself both to its own different aspects of personality and to Jung's idea of the collective unconscious. Sessions are either conducted on a one-to-one basis or, quite often, in groups or workshops. Guided imagery, meditation, dream work, drawing and painting are often used and therapists frequently focus on unblocking the chakras, the Eastern energy centres of the body.

WOMEN'S THERAPY (FEMINIST THERAPY): This is based on the recognition that women have three common issues: autonomy or power, self-nurturing and anger. In women's therapy, women are encouraged to direct anger, to confront the restrictions placed on them and to learn to look after themselves, as well as others. It often incorporates elements of Gestalt, transactional analysis and client-centred therapy.

Self-counselling – the basic plan

This is a very condensed version of an outline for self-counselling. You will need to find a time and place where you won't be disturbed. Allow yourself a clear, uninterrupted hour for each session. Take a break of a week between each session.

SESSION ONE Focus on what you want to achieve.
- First, write down the changes you want to make – whatever comes into your mind. If it feels more comfortable, speak them into a tape recorder before copying them onto paper.
- Now go over your account and notice the kind of language you have used. Change negative phrases to positive ones – e.g. rather than say 'I want to stop smoking', phrase it as 'I will become a non-smoker'. 'I won't be so unassertive' could be 'I will stand up for my rights'. Make sure your changes are clear and measurable – make your goals very precise.
- Check your goal doesn't depend on other people changing. You can never guarantee a change in other people – the only person over whom you have that kind of control is yourself.
- Do you know anyone who has achieved what you want? He or she could give valuable advice or provide a good example.
- Think about how you will actually be different when you have achieved your desired change. Define in detail what you and others will be able to see and hear you doing differently. Be very specific. Check that the changes you are contemplating are safe for you. Think through the results of any changes you want to make. If you became more assertive with your employer, for example, you might lose your job. Are you ready and willing to risk making the changes you want? Is the change really for you? Make sure you are seeking to change for your own benefit.
- Return to your original statement. You may want to rewrite it in the light of your answers to the previous questions.

SESSION TWO Look at what is happening in your life now.

• What is actually happening to me now? (Be specific – keep to what is happening, rather than what you think may be happening.) What is not happening? What are other people doing or not doing? Now ask what you are thinking. It is important to distinguish between thought, feeling and action. What are you feeling? What are you doing? What would you prefer to be happening? What would you be doing if you were succeeding? What are you willing to do to start? How is that different from what you are actually doing? What is the worst thing that could happen? How might you sabotage yourself?

• Listen to the language that you have used. Is it vague? Make it precise. Are your problems based on fact or on how you perceive the situation? Be honest with yourself.

SESSION THREE Write your life script. This may well help you gain insight into your behaviour and feelings in the present.

• What is your earliest memory? Is there a family story about your birth? How were you named? Describe your parents. Describe yourself. What was your parents' advice to you? What did they want you to be? What made them angry with you? How did they express their anger? What do you like most, and least, about yourself? What do you wish your parents had done differently? If, by magic, you could change anything about yourself, for what would you wish? What do you want most out of life? Do you think of yourself as a winner or a loser? What will it say on your tombstone?

• Can you see any patterns emerging? Are there any attitudes or beliefs from the past that are affecting you in the present? The script can give important clues – you may be able to see clear connections between your present ways of thinking, feeling and behaving, and the early decisions you made.

SESSION FOUR Resolving differences. At this stage, there is a variety of different techniques and approaches you can use to help you leave the past behind and move forwards to make the changes you desire. Sometimes just recognizing where thoughts and beliefs come from can provide a breakthrough, but often you will need to do more work. One suggestion is to use the 'empty chair' of Gestalt therapy. This is very useful if the earlier sessions have shown that you have 'unfinished business' with anyone in your life (either alive or dead).

• Set up your room so you are sitting opposite an empty chair or floor cushion. Imagine the person to whom you want to speak is sitting in the chair. Voice what you want him or her to hear.

• When you have finished having your say, move to the empty chair yourself and pretend you are the other person. Let him or her speak through you – the response may be very predictable or you may be surprised by what you say or feel.

• Let the conversation continue – switching chairs as necessary – until you are satisfied that you have said all you wish. Now sit quietly and reflect on any insights you have gained.

4 Swift Solutions

While many of the 'talking therapies' can demand a long commitment, a new breed of psychotherapies aims to give a quick yet effective fix. These strategies can be surprisingly powerful and are certainly worth a try if you feel that standard psychotherapy is not for you.

Solution therapy

Traditional therapies usually take months (and sometimes years) to see results, but brief therapy, or solution-focused therapy (to give it its full name), will often dispatch people after one or two sessions. It may seem incredible, yet the changes that can occur following that short spell can appear truly miraculous, with effects that can last forever.

The new wonder therapy was developed in the USA by researcher Steve De Shazer. He discovered that, despite the common concept of psychotherapy needing to be a long-term process, in actual fact people attended an average of only seven sessions. If they could get what they needed so quickly, he reasoned, surely a new model could be developed that expected and facilitated rapid results. The result was initially called brief therapy, but many now prefer the title solution-focused therapy, or simply solution therapy.

While standard therapists and analysts will spend hours looking at your 'problem', solution therapists are not really interested in how your life isn't working. Instead of focusing on the problem, solution therapists look at the time when the problem does not exist. Say you have a panic attack that lasts for an hour. Normal therapy would probably focus on that one hour, whereas solution therapists are interested in the 23 hours of the day when the panic attack didn't happen. In other words, you have strategies that stop you from having panic attacks all day long and the solution therapist would want to find out what they were and how you could continue the strategies to cover that one stray hour.

Central to solution therapy is the idea that, even before we come to therapy, we have methods in place for coping with our problems. The therapist is not there to instruct, but to encourage us to believe in our innate problem-solving facility.

What can solution therapy help?

- It has proved successful for anxiety problems, those who suffer depression and even for people with severe addictions.
- Survivors of abuse frequently benefit and the model is also of immense help in family and couple therapy.
- Solution therapy could help you stop smoking or lose weight.

- This therapy is about crisis resolution, rather than personal growth. It's good for people who want a quick resolution, but not those who want to explore feelings or look into the past.

What can I expect from a session?

WHERE WILL I HAVE THE SESSION?
You will be sitting in a room with (usually) two or more therapists.

WILL I BE CLOTHED?
Yes, you will be fully clothed.

WHAT HAPPENS?
First, therapists will ask clients why they have come and how they would like them to help. Then, as early as possible, they ask what they call the 'miracle question': 'If you woke up one day and your life was exactly how you wanted it to be, how would you know?' Naturally, most people's first response is something like 'I would feel better', 'I would have won the lottery' or 'My husband would still be alive' – seemingly impossible daydreams, foolish wish fulfilment. However, out of these dreams, the therapists may uncover perfectly realistic goals. By careful questioning, the team will find out precisely what winning the lottery, for example, may mean. The questioning continues to build up a solid map of behavioural changes – some large, some very small. It's the small and insignificant that solution therapists suggest form the first steps of change. When you achieve them, you will have the motivation and encouragement to take the next step, and the next, and so on.

WILL IT HURT?
No, this is not a painful therapy – either physically or emotionally.

WILL ANYTHING STRANGE HAPPEN?
No, solution therapy is very down-to-earth and practical.

WILL I BE GIVEN ANYTHING TO TAKE?
No, medication is not part of the treatment.

IS THERE ANY HOMEWORK?
Yes, you will be asked to make initially very small shifts in your life.

Mapping miracles – solution therapy

Solution therapy can be ideal when you want simply to resolve a problem or crisis, rather than delve deeply into your psyche for weeks on end. If you are in need of crisis resolution, try asking the following questions.
1 If you woke up and all your problems and worries had disappeared, how would you know a miracle had happened?
2 How would you behave differently? (Be as precise as possible.)
3 How would your family and friends behave differently?
4 How do you think your family and friends would know a miracle had happened? How would they see the differences in you and your behaviour?
5 Are there parts of the miracle that are already happening in your life?

6 How have you made these things happen? Is it possible for you to make more of them happen?

7 What elements of your life at present would you like to continue?

8 On a scale of nought to ten, where nought is the worst your life has been and ten is the day after the miracle, where are you now?

9 If you are on, say, four, how would you get to five? What would you be doing differently?

10 How would your family know you had moved up one point?

NLP – the master communicator

What makes one person succeed where another fails? How is it that some people can debate metaphysics in a foreign language, while the rest of us still stumble over 'Two beers, please'? Are we simply genetically wired to be either superachievers or also-rans, or can we change the program? The advocates of neuro-linguistic programming (NLP) insist that there's a swift, scientific, precise technique that will stop you languishing in the mire of mediocrity – we can, they insist, all become superpeople. If one person in the world can do it, according to NLP, so can you – you just need to learn precisely how they do it and then copy them. This is a technique called 'modelling', which can, if properly applied, give us a precise map to achieve the same excellence as the person we model.

NLP started in the 1970s in California, when Richard Bandler (a mathematician and Gestalt therapist) and John Grinder (a professor of linguistics) began to question exactly what made some people brilliant in their work, while others remained mediocre. They selected three acknowledged experts in the field of therapy and 'modelled' them, finding out exactly how they worked, how they thought, how they perceived, how they moved and spoke, what minute processes took place and precisely the sequence in which they happened. Their findings led to NLP: not really a therapy, more a precise tool for understanding human communication and improving it – a way of working out what causes excellence and how we can each achieve it. Bandler and Grinder swiftly went on to model athletes, dancers, teachers, businesspeople, even politicians. The results were so impressive that they put their findings together and called this system for analysing excellence NLP. It's like taking an advanced driving course – but for living.

The first lesson is that, in order to communicate effectively with someone, you have to know which 'mode' they are in. We have three modes of functioning – visual, auditory and kinaesthetic (feeling) – and you can usually tell which mode a person is using at any given time by their body posture, the speed of their speech, their breathing and even the words they use (see page 30). NLP teaches that much of our misunderstanding arises when people communicate in different modes – when a person in visual mode tries to communicate with someone in an auditory state, for example. Good communicators 'match' the person they are talking to, so if they are talking to a 'visual' person, they, too, will go into visual mode, speaking rapidly, breathing quite high in the chest and using 'visual' words and phrases such as 'I look at it this way', 'I see what you mean' or 'What's the overall picture?' Suddenly you are speaking the same language.

Following on from this is rapport building, in which, by subtly mirroring the person we are talking to (adopting a similar posture/speaking at the same speed/breathing in synchronization), we can almost instantly put someone at ease.

Basically, it is all about learning how brains work and how different people's brains work in different ways. Simple techniques can prove highly effective in any situation, from soothing the boss or getting through to the kids, to communicating honestly with your partner.

Understanding how brains work is also fundamental to the ability to model. In order to copy someone exactly, it's not enough merely to mimic their physical moves, you have to get inside their head, to find out the processes behind an action. If, say, you wanted to model an expert skier, you might first watch his or her technique very carefully. You might move your body in the same motions as you watch, until they feel like a part of you. Next, you would make an internal picture of an expert skiing, then conjure up a disassociated image of yourself skiing – like watching a film of yourself modelling the other person as precisely as possible. Next, you would step inside that picture and experience how it would feel to perform the same action precisely the way the expert athlete did. You would repeat this as often as it would take for you to feel completely comfortable doing it. This strategy, say NLP practitioners, could give you the specific neurological strategy that could help you perform at optimum levels. Then you would try it in the real world.

Are you visual, auditory or kinaesthetic?

NLP teaches that we each favour a specific 'pathway' or mode of perceiving the world – visual, auditory or kinaesthetic. But how can you tell?

- Have someone ask you a question that requires you to recollect something in the past, e.g. what did you do last weekend? If, when you answer, you look up to the other person's right, you are predominantly visual. If your eyes slide from the left to the right of their face, you are mainly auditory. If you look down and to the left then right before answering, you are working in a kinaesthetic pathway.
- How do you best learn a new subject? Do you memorize a page of information (visual), repeat facts out loud (auditory) or write down what you are learning (kinaesthetic)?
- What kinds of words do you use to express yourself? Do you talk in terms of seeing ('I see what you mean', 'The picture is clear', 'Look at me when I'm talking to you'): all primarily visual. Or do you talk in terms of hearing ('I hear what you're saying', 'I'd like to sound them out', 'Listen to me when I'm talking to you'): auditory. Or do you express yourself in terms of feeling ('I feel it in my bones', 'It really touched me', 'Can't you feel the difference?'): kinaesthetic.
- If you're assessing children, there are other ways of gauging which mode they use. When they are angry, do they look you in the eye with defiance (visual), scream and shout (auditory), or stamp their feet or throw themselves to the ground (kinaesthetic)? What would they notice first on a walk in the park? Other children, the birds and animals around (visual); the sound of music playing, dogs barking or people shouting (auditory), or the wind, the rain, the cold or the heat (kinaesthetic)?

This all sounds very interesting in theory, but what help is it practically? Well, if you decided to learn a new language, it would be helpful to choose a method that allowed you to work in your most comfortable pathway. A series of audio tapes would not be enough for a kinaesthetic person, while an auditory person would not do so well with a simple textbook. A visual person will always manage better with clear text and diagrams, an auditory person through spoken words and a kinaesthetic with practical examples. In an ideal learning situation, all three pathways will be used.

NLP can also help you to understand people and to communicate better. People find that they get on much better with their boss or a difficult member of their family if they can talk the same language, picking up on which pathway the person works in and shifting their language to match that person. It's subtle but highly effective and, if you are interested in good communication, well worth investigating in greater depth.

Swish technique – turning past failure into present success

The swish technique from NLP offers a swift way to change negative patterns of behaviour. It is often used to help people overcome fears and phobias – such as of public speaking or flying – or handle difficult situations better, so they can prevent habitual arguments, cope with a difficult boss, become more assertive.

1 Identify the behaviour you want to change. Close your eyes and decide on a cue picture. This is what you might see, hear and feel just before you start the behaviour that you want to change. So, for example, it might be you feeling and looking small and unimportant.

2 Now create a picture of how you would like to look and feel and sound instead – if you were to be in your ideal, confident, energized state. Make the picture really clear and really powerful. You should feel a little shiver of energy when the picture's just right.

3 Now imagine your unpleasant cue picture is on a huge movie screen. It's big, clear and in full colour. It should be pretty unpleasant to see.

4 Now place the picture of the new confident you on the screen, down in the bottom left-hand corner. Make this picture small and in black and white.

5 Now you can start 'swishing'. Imagine the small positive picture zooming up to fill the whole screen, completely obliterating the negative picture. As the picture expands, it becomes bright, multicoloured and clear. In contrast, the negative picture shrinks away into a corner, gradually becoming small and dark.

6 Open your eyes, stamp your feet and shake your arms out. Clear your mind of the picture.

7 Now repeat the procedure (steps 4 and 5) as quickly as possible, stopping and blanking the screen in your mind's eye between each swish.

You can boost your confidence by swishing just before you have to go into any difficult situation. The difference it makes should be enormous.

Timeline therapy

Timeline is a precise, swift technique which developed out of NLP. By changing your relationship with time, you can transform your whole life. Timeline therapy teaches that the only difference between people who just dream and the people who live their dreams is that the people who live their dreams do something different with their thinking. At a deep, subconscious level, they truly believe things will happen.

Make time work for you

You may find it easier to practise these exercises with a partner guiding you. Sit down comfortably in a chair and relax. Some people may find it easier to close their eyes.

FINDING YOUR TIMELINE: Have someone give you the following prompts. As you think about the time in question, you will find you access the information in a particular place in your mind's eye (e.g. up to the left, down to the right, over to the side). If you find it hard to work out where you are holding time, have your partner observe your body language. You may indicate where the thought is held by a movement of the hand, the eyes or your head.

- Think of something you might be doing in 3 months.
- Think of something you might be doing in 3 years.
- Think of where you might be 10 years down the line.
- Think of something that happened last week.
- Think of something that happened 6 months ago.
- Think of something that happened 5 years ago.

Pay attention to where your thoughts are. See if you can draw a line between them. It might go from side to side, forwards and backwards, or be quite convoluted. This is your timeline. Become used to it – imagine where events lie on it.

Make your dreams come true

Think about something you really want to happen. Now make your dream as specific as you can.

- Ask yourself: 'What is the last thing that has to happen for me to know that I have achieved my dream?' What would you need to see, to hear, to feel, to know you've achieved it?
- Really imagine that scene. See it in clear detail. Make it just right, as perfect as it can be, as real as it can be.
- Step slightly out of the picture, but keep it clearly in your mind's eye. The emotional intensity will feel slightly less, but that's fine. Freeze-frame the picture, like a snapshot.
- Rise up way above your timeline, imagining it stretching out below. Hold the picture with you and imagine you're floating out above the future. Now let the picture go; let it float down onto the timeline, onto the right time for your dream to become reality. Watch it settle on the line and watch all the events between then and now realigning themselves to support your outcome.
- When you are ready, float back to the present.

You have now set your subconscious to 'create' the future for you. But remember you might still have to put in some effort. Timeline will create the opportunities – you have to take them.

5 Work Harmony

How many of us, hands on heart, are in jobs that we really love? Doubtless the answer is very few. Yet our work is how we spend the majority of our waking lives. Doesn't it therefore seem more than a little strange that we are quite resigned to the fact that work is usually a drag? That work should be hard, difficult and relatively unpleasant? Earning money must, by its very definition, be something serious. But why? Why shouldn't we enjoy our work?

Work takes up such a hefty chunk of our lives that it seems criminal to continue with a job that makes us truly unhappy. Few of us take the time to analyse precisely why we do the work we do and where exactly the problems lie. We often make career decisions in haste, in panic, at the drop of a hat. Although you may insist that you hate your job, it is worth sitting down and asking exactly what it is you hate about it. It may well be only one element of your work that you dislike. Armed with that knowledge, you are in a much better position to decide whether to do the same work in a new company, to alter the kind of work you do in the same organization or to change both your job and your company.

You do have a choice. The trouble is that we often end up in a job through force of circumstance and then believe that we can't change. Why not, though, fit what you enjoy being good at with the ideal career? By analysing precisely what constitutes your 'job personality', you can make your working life more profitable, more involving and much more fun.

It's worth setting aside a day, or a couple of evenings, to work solely on yourself and your career. It is vital to give yourself your undivided attention. Before you start, try to get into a relaxed state. Take some deep breaths, stretch, roll your neck slowly round. Detach yourself from your normal tasks and commitments. Don't look on these exercises as a chore. Pretend it's a game; have fun and feel free to use coloured crayons, paints or huge pieces of paper – whatever appeals. If you want to draw pictures, that's great.

Above all, be honest. Remember, no one needs to see this except you. Put down everything you can think of, however silly or unrelated it may appear. Some people have forged incredible careers by unearthing skills and pleasures in things they did at school or at a youth club.

Our family script

We acquire many of our deep-seated beliefs about work at a very young age from previous generations for whom the concept of work was often intrinsically bound up with notions of duty, discipline and hard slog. Consequently, we are almost all following other people's work scripts, obeying decisions we made almost subconsciously before we even entered the workplace. By becoming aware of your scripts, you can let go of a large number of preconceptions about the nature of work, about the kind of job you are in and about your expectations.

- Ask yourself your thoughts about work. For example, do you think: 'I never get what I really want'; 'I have to fight and be tough to make myself heard'; 'I have to have a "proper" professional career, like a doctor or lawyer'?
- Write down whatever comes to mind, however silly it may seem. Spend some time pondering where those thoughts originated. Did you feel dissatisfied at school, perhaps? Or was your father never promoted beyond a certain level? Did your parents tell you how much your education was costing and that you owed it to them to get a 'sensible' job?
- Look at your thoughts logically. Decide whether they are appropriate for you now. If not, be willing to let them go. Merely by being aware of your internal script, you can reassess your work pattern.

Finding your job personality

Realizing that most of your conclusions about the kind of work you should be doing are based on other people's decisions means you can now look at what you really want.

- Make an audit of all your skills, your knowledge, your attributes and qualities, your hobbies. Start from as early as you like and put down everything that you can think of. Include the subjects you learnt at school and college; the jobs and careers that you have had and the qualities and skills they called for; the extracurricular activities and hobbies you enjoyed; and any workshops or training.
- Don't judge what you are writing – for example, don't think, 'Acting in school plays is irrelevant to me as an accountant.' Everything is important, from playing in the softball team to enjoying caring for your younger siblings.
- Decide which are your favourite three skills. Flesh out each skill with stories from your past: how you used this skill, what the situation was, who was there, how it felt. Can you think of any skills you enjoyed using on lots of occasions? Say you like organizing: be very precise about how exactly you enjoy organizing. Do you enjoy organizing people or data or things? Do you enjoy organizing in a methodical, logical way or using your intuition and gut reactions? Were you part of a team, managing the team or working alone?
- Look at your stories and decide which are your favourites.

You will now have a good idea of where your skills and areas of expertise lie. You may well feel you would like to develop a skill or start using an old skill again. You might consider that your present job really doesn't represent your true skills and breadth of knowledge. Jot down any thoughts that come into your head and then move on.

The ideal workplace

Your present job might already be using all your skills and knowledge, but you are still unhappy. The trouble could well be where you are working. Once you know what your skills are, you must question the context in which you want to use them.

- Look back at your audit and make a list of the environments in which you have either worked or learnt. For each stage of your life, ask yourself about the kind of organization you were in: was it large or small, public or private sector? What did it produce (did it make things, disseminate information, help people, etc.)? Was the workforce primarily male, female, or mixed? Did you work alone, in a small team, as part of a large structure? Note any patterns. Were you always happiest working primarily on your own, but reporting to a small group of co-workers? Do you like to be part of a large, organized team involved in caring?
- Ask yourself what you really want from a workplace. Do you like working for established businesses; for new, growing concerns; for non-profit-making organizations? Do you like working for an organization that manufactures things (if so, what kind of things?); one that processes information (how do you like to deal with information?); or one that works with people (exactly what kind of people? What age range, what background? Individuals or groups? Easygoing or difficult people?).
- Would you be happy if you changed your work environment? For instance, instead of teaching large groups of adults, would you like to give one-to-one help to children with special needs? Would you rather be working for a small, personal company than an established, large, safe firm? Maybe you simply need to change the way you work. If you are lonely working on your own, perhaps you could become part of a team or work under the auspices of a larger department which would give support and feedback.

Your work language

Lots of people have discovered that they enjoy the skills they use, but hate the language they have to speak. Yet a solicitor does not have to speak just 'solicitese': she could also speak the language of film or theatre, of medicine, of psychology, or of shipping, depending on the environment in which she pursues her skills. An administrator might love his job, might feel very happy with the size and structure of the organization for which he works, but hate the fact that it deals in military uniforms because, over the past few years, his views on defence have fundamentally changed. You can never be happy in a job if you wince every time you hear certain words or phrases.
- Look at your subject list, your list of areas of knowledge, and highlight any that you couldn't stand working with all day long. Which are your favourites? Which would you be happy talking about and hearing about all day long?

Creating your ideal job

You should now have most of the information you require to discover your ideal work situation. Pull it all together and find the anatomy of your ideal job.
- Think about anything you might have missed in the previous exercises. Ask yourself what your dreams are – if this were the last day of your life, what would you regret not ever having done? Incorporate any answers into your job anatomy.
- Indulge in some playful thinking around matching your favourite things to possible jobs. Be inventive, be silly, don't analyse. Think of ways to link even the most incongruous qualities: use it as a test of your lateral thinking.

Making links

Now is the time to start thinking about the external factors: what is out there and how to match what employers want with what you have to offer. Don't immediately fly to the nearest employment agency or job advertisements. People who think in unorthodox patterns stand far more chance of success. If you reply to an advertisement in a newspaper, your odds are pretty slim – you could be competing against hundreds of applicants. If you go for a job from an employment agency, you will still be up against a fair few. But if you target a specific organization and convince its personnel that you are tailor-made for it, you are competing against nobody. Yes, you might argue, but there is no vacancy. Perhaps not, but people who know precisely what they want and match their skills to a specific organization often prove irresistible.

- Spend some time asking yourself the following questions. Which of my skills could be used in a variety of occupations? Which jobs would allow me to use my favourite skills in a field based on my favourite subjects or areas of knowledge?
- Which organizations or companies employ people in these roles? Which of these organizations do I like? Which of these organizations need my skills and knowledge?
- Ask friends or family to give some input. Show them your list of criteria and see if they have any thoughts or hunches.

The core statement

If you prefer a more unusual approach to career appraisal, try the core statement. It's a clever technique which helps people discover the kind of role in life that could make their 'soul sing'. It has put frustrated businesspeople back in the fast lane and helped firms build teams of highly motivated workers. It can give absolutely everybody a clear insight into what really makes them tick – and tick joyously.

The core statement is, very simply, a clear, concise statement of your life's purpose. It outlines the criteria that have to be fulfilled in order to keep you contented and committed to your path in life – to make you adore your days, rather than just get by. Composing it rarely takes more than an hour and, once you have it, you have it for life.

All of us have quite specific roles that we feel happiest playing in life. While one person may relish new challenges, another may love nothing better than the safe and secure. Where one person thrives working alone, another may feel lost without the support and stimulus of a team or family.

Our core statement tends to be clearest in childhood, before we succumb to the pressures of school and work. It's as if there were a line of arrows leading through our lives that shows where we should be going. Unfortunately, many of us veer away from that path – as a result of pressure at school or college, or in the workplace. Also, while most of us think that our daily grind is simply something to endure, people who practise the core-statement philosophy point out that such an attitude could be positively injurious to our health and happiness. When the gap between what we should be doing and what we are doing becomes too great, we start to become stressed and eventually even sick.

To be happy and efficient, we need to be working in the right environment, in the right way or with the right people. Sometimes all you need is a small adjustment to make all the difference. The process itself is simple, yet also great fun. It requires you to look back over your life and pinpoint the times when you were utterly enthralled by life, totally absorbed or totally exhilarated.

It isn't always practical to do precisely what you want. Life is not perfect, but you can get within a certain bandwidth. If you can't be totally fulfilled at work, you need to compensate for that by doing what you love in your leisure time.

Finding your core statement

You can start to understand what makes you 'sing your song' by thinking about the following. Work with another person, as he or she may notice which phrases are stressed or repeated.

1 Find a joyful childhood memory. Have your partner ask you the following: 'What were you doing?', 'What made it special?', 'How did you feel?', 'Was anyone with you?', 'What did you enjoy the most?' Write down the key phrases and words.

2 Think of a good time in your life, at any period. Repeat the questions and again write down key phrases or words.

3 Repeat the above process with the following:
   • talk about a fulfilling work experience
   • explore a hobby or pastime
   • capture a moment when you felt complete.

4 Now identify the most important key phrases and words and write them down on paper. Which keep recurring? Where are the patterns? Which represent the most important circumstances or attitudes? If you could have only three or four of these phrases or words, which would they be?

5 Try to compose a sentence that incorporates these phrases and has real meaning for you. When you hit on the right statement, it will instinctively feel right – some people laugh or even cry. Play with words until yours emerges.

Using feng shui in the workplace

Just as feng shui can make a difference to your home life, it can be very important at work as well. Many big corporations now insist on having feng shui consultants analyse their workplaces for the best possible flow of qi, vital energy. You, too, can take advantage of this subtle energy to make your workplace more pleasant and your career more successful. There are simple guidelines for success and happy working conditions in the office.

• Your desk should always be positioned diagonally opposite the door, with you facing the door. You need to be able to see everyone who walks into your office the moment they enter. This makes good sense psychologically (no one can creep up on you and surprise you), but is also said to be the 'power position' that will give you control, concentration and a sense of natural authority.

• Computer workers who have their backs to the door will become stressed. According to feng shui, sitting with your back to the door, whatever your job, can even cause you to be demoted or made redundant. If, for whatever reason, you really can't change your desk position, put up a mirror so that you can see people approaching. Mirrors can also be used in offices to draw in money-endowing water views (if your office looks out over any kind of water, make sure a mirror reflects the view). Water is considered to equate with wealth and success. What happens if your desk is immovable and your

boss frowns on the idea of mirrors? Slip a mirror into your desk drawer facing the desired direction, as a symbolic protection.
- If you are the boss, make sure you don't sit too close to the door of your office, particularly if other workers or secretaries share it with you. If you do, you will be treated as an underling and lose respect. Workers in better and more advantageous spots will become insubordinate.
- If you work for a difficult boss and you have to sit directly in front of or behind him or her, be sure to place either a crystal paperweight or a bowl of water on your desk. It will deflect any criticism or intolerance. If you can put goldfish in your bowl, even better.
- Watch out for workers who sit close to the door. They tend to leave early and avoid overtime. A mirror positioned to take the worker's attention away from the door will cure this.
- If you can, incorporate a fish tank into your office, preferably positioned in the wealth corner. A tank with a bubbling aerator is most effective. Ideally, you should have eight red fish and one black one.

Feng shui your desk

Your desk is the key to success at work. Whether you want a better relationship with your boss or a nice fat raise, you need to use the art of feng shui to boost your opportunities. Where you place your desk and what you place on it can make the difference between make or break in business – be you a big boss in a corporate office or self-employed in a corner of your living room. Ideally, your desk should be positioned so you are sitting with your back against a solid wall with a good view of both the door and the window. Above all, make sure you keep your desk free of clutter: if your desk is buried under a pile of paperwork, it will make you feel tired and depressed before you start your day. Here's how to arrange your desk to boost your career.
- Keep a bright, functional desk lamp on one side of your desk – this helps to hold your attention. Place it on the far left-hand side of your desk to improve your finances. If you would rather increase your recognition, put it directly in front of you. If you need to get on better with people, place it in the top right-hand corner.
- Fresh-cut flowers stimulate mental activity and cleanse the atmosphere. The colour and number of flowers are important: four red or purple flowers in a vase will help boost your income; two yellow flowers in the top right-hand corner will help you get on with people. In general, flowers will boost your creativity and recognition.
- Your telephone can sit in either the bottom left-hand or bottom right-hand corner of your desk. The right side is ideal, as it will make people more helpful when you call them. If you are left-handed, keep your address book on your right instead to gain a similar result.
- Keep essential reference books on your left-hand side, the knowledge area.
- Opposite your desk, make sure you have something that stimulates your creativity or reminds you of your goals.
- If your work is creative, try to have a rounded desk. If your work involves figures or is very precise, a square desk is better, but ideally still with rounded corners.
- Try to use a square briefcase or handbag to make you more inclined to complete projects.
- When cheques come in, put them in the top left-hand corner of your desk, perhaps weighted down by a beautiful paperweight. Place your invoices here, too, before you send them out.

- If you work in a team or want to get on better with your colleagues, put a photograph of your work team in the top right-hand corner of your desk. Place a candle in front of it to boost the good energy.

Getting on with people

Sometimes the hardest thing about a job is the people with whom we work. When a crowd of people work together in close proximity, it's understandable that not everyone will get on all the time. Recognizing that we are all very different can help. There are also some interesting techniques that can help head off problems and resolve any conflicts that do emerge.

Revisit the information on NLP (pages 29–31). Be aware of how your colleagues view the world and, if you find yourself slipping into disagreement, try using their language to make them feel less threatened and more understood.

If you find yourself in a difficult situation, with an argument brewing, try the following tactics.

- First of all, say: 'Let's have a 5-minute break and come back to this.' A pause will allow both/all of you to calm down and rethink. Use this time to go somewhere quiet and to work through these suggestions.
- Take a few minutes to sit calmly and breathe deeply. Feel yourself breathing out the anger and irritation, and breathing in new ideas and responses.
- Write down the reasons for the disagreement. Pour out all your feelings of anger and irritation onto paper (it may be a good idea to write an imaginary letter to the person or people). This can help release the negative emotions safely and also put things in perspective.
- Try seeing the other point of view. If you find this hard (or even downright impossible!), the empty-chair technique from Gestalt therapy is useful (see page 22). Sit on one chair and imagine the other person sitting on the other. Describe exactly how you feel. Now swap chairs and imagine you are the other person. Put yourself in his or her shoes and talk to the other chair as if you were the other person talking to you. What might he or she be thinking, feeling? What might he or she really want to say? Swap chairs again, continuing the conversation (or argument) for as long as it takes to understand both sides of the question (there always are two sides to every question).
- Take two drops of beech flower remedy under your tongue. Beech will help you stop being overcritical and angry. If your colleague(s) will take some, too, so much the better.
- When you return to the other person or people, visualize love and understanding flowing from your heart chakra towards others. You may like to visualize it as a beautiful pink-gold bubble of unconditional love. Although this may be difficult, do try your best!

6 Home Harmony

If your home is piled high with clutter and mess, you will never feel comfortable and relaxed in it. On a physical level, clutter attracts dust and cobwebs. In energetic terms, it prevents qi from circulating freely – the energy stagnates. Psychologists also believe that, when we are surrounded by confusion, our minds become equally confused and anxious.

Decluttering is the first step that any feng shui (see pages 42–3) consultant will advise you to take and it will make an enormous difference to your feeling of wellbeing. The Chinese believe that, when we get rid of the old, it allows room for something new to take its place – an idea worth holding on to if you find it hard to let go!

How you clear the clutter is up to you. Some people like to have an enormous clear-out, going through the whole house like a whirlwind and filling an entire skip! Others will need to take it more slowly, maybe focusing on a different room (or even just a drawer) each week.

Decluttering your home

1   Set aside a specific time for decluttering your home. Make it fun: put on some favourite music; burn some aromatherapy oils (something fresh and stimulating such as lemon, grapefruit or pine). If you know that you'll be overcome with nostalgia, take some clematis Bach flower remedy. Promise yourself a treat at the end of your decluttering (even if it's just a glass of freshly squeezed juice or a cup of herbal tea – and a magazine).

2   If you have loads of other people's stuff, put it all in a box and ask them to come and collect it. Say you're having a clear-out and that anything remaining after, say, a month, will be donated to charity.

3   If you have a family heirloom that you really don't want, offer it to other members of the family. If no one wants it, agree to sell it and have a family outing with the proceeds. Don't be guilt-tripped into keeping it!

4   Nearly new clothes and expensive mistakes can go to dress agencies, or be given to friends. Take any unwanted clean, serviceable clothes to charity outlets.

5   Furniture and unwanted (working) electrical goods can be advertised in your local newspaper (often for free or a small fee). Otherwise, charities for the elderly and disabled people will often come and collect them.

6   Donate magazines to hospitals or your doctor's/dentist's/vet's surgery. Clip out any newspaper cuttings you need and put them in a book, then recycle your newspapers and other clean paper products.

7   Keep an 'essential papers' file for your important documents. Keep sentimental letters and keepsakes in a beautiful box. Put important contact details in an address book, personal organizer or on a computer disk. Then let go of all the other papers: recycle or have a bonfire!

8   Old medicines can be dangerous; old cosmetics can go rancid. Safely dispose of old medicines (usually to your pharmacist) and dump cosmetics older than a year.

9   It's not hygienic to use chipped or cracked crockery. Use it to make mosaics if you're artistic; otherwise, put it in the garbage (trash).

10 Weed out your book and record collection and sell any unwanted items to second-hand stores or give them to charity outlets or jumble sales.

The smell-good home

Scent is another way to make your home harmonious with a minimum of effort. Change the smell of your home and you can shift its atmosphere and mood from soothing sanctuary to vibrant party place whenever you wish. However, don't be tempted by artificial fragrances and air fresheners: synthetic smells are a common trigger for asthma and hayfever. Instead, seek out pure aromatherapy products. Use them in a fragrance burner, add them to a bath or fill bowls with warm water and add a few drops to scent a room gently (place on a radiator to release the odour over a longer time).

The following are the best oils for starting – but don't use aromatherapy products if you are pregnant, unless you consult a trained aromatherapist first.

• Geranium lifts your mood – use it if you're feeling down or to welcome guests into your home.
• Lavender is wonderful for deep relaxation.
• Lemon is uplifting. Put a few drops in the washing-up liquid.
• Peppermint is energizing, but can increase your appetite (so avoid if you're trying to lose weight!).
• Rosemary can help concentration – burn some on your desk as you work.
• Ylang ylang is sensuous and sexy! Use it whenever you want to bring romance and passion into your life.

Colours for the home

Colour has the power to lift our spirits, to soothe our souls, to enliven us or calm us. By bringing colour into your home, you can subtly but very effectively change the atmosphere of the house. See colour therapy (pages 67–9) for more ideas.

• Ideally, your bedroom should always tend towards the cooler hues – soft blues, greens and mauves, which will slow down the brain and soothe the nervous system. But do incorporate some vibrant red or pink (in the form of cushions or throws) if you want to liven up your sex life!
• Pick warm shades for kitchens and living rooms. Colour therapists say that pink or peach encourages people to draw closer together, share feelings and discuss them. Pink also helps people to relax, let go, unwind and feel at ease; it dispels stress and tension. Orange, yellow and apricot are equally suitable. Orange, in particular, is a very sociable colour – ideal for living rooms where people congregate.

- Soft indigo or violet are wonderful if you have a meditation or retreat room. They can also be soothing for guest rooms.
- If you live in a studio apartment or have to double up your living and sleeping space, go for soft greens – they are soothing enough for sleep, yet comfortable for daytime, too.

Feng shui

Feng shui evolved around 5,000 years ago in China. The ancient Chinese believed that invisible life energy (known as qi, or chi) flowed through everything in life. It's the same philosophy that underlies acupuncture – if the energy in your body is moving freely and easily, you will stay fit and healthy. Should it become stagnant or blocked, however, you will most likely fall ill. In acupuncture, needles are used to free any blockages and to regulate the smooth flowing of qi. The principle is much the same in houses and offices, but various 'cures' are used instead of needles.

The Chinese believed that the buildings we live and work in require quite as much attention as our bodies; as a result, they developed this complex science for 'healing' our environment. Centuries of observation suggested to them that different areas of the house or room attracted specific energies. Furthermore, the Chinese believed that certain configurations (the layout of rooms or even the position of furniture or features) could either help or hinder the free, smooth flowing of energy. If the energy was blocked or allowed to flow too swiftly, it would cause corresponding blockages and problems in life. Fortunately, however, they realized that very small but specific changes ('cures' such as hanging wind chimes or crystals in particular places or using certain colours) could correct such disharmony and put a life back on track. Augmenting particular areas with auspicious colours and objects could even create better energy and hence better opportunities in life.

At its core, the philosophy of feng shui teaches that, by making small shifts to your home, you can affect everything in your life – from your finances to your health, and even your marriage and sex life.

Although feng shui sounds mystical, it is taken very seriously, not just in its native China but all over the world.

Mapping your home

One of the fundamental principles of feng shui is in the *ba-gua*. This is an imaginary octagonal template that divides any space (your entire house, an apartment or office or simply a room) into eight areas (or corners). These represent wealth, fame, marriage, children, helpful people, career, knowledge and the family. In order to work out the *ba-gua* of any room or house, the position of the main door is important. If it lies in the middle of your wall, it is in the position known as career. If it is to the left of centre, it is in the position known as knowledge, and if it is to the right, it is in the position known as helpful people. Imagine yourself standing with your back to the door with the *ba-gua* laid over your space. Then work your way clockwise around the room.

You can apply the *ba-gua* to any building or room. Having worked out what lies where in your house, you can often see whence your problems may be emanating. Not all houses are built perfectly square and symmetrical – often you will find you are missing an area of the *ba-gua*. An L-shaped house might well be missing the marriage area. Equally, the marriage area in your bedroom might be the place where you keep a cluttered desk or the dirty laundry. Neither of these would help your relationships because the qi would become stagnant and heavy. If money is a problem, make sure your wealth area is clean and clear (and maybe add a feature such as a water fountain or fish tank to boost finances).

Resolving qi problems

Fortunately, there are umpteen very simple 'cures' used in feng shui that can help resolve problems in your home's qi. They are generally cheap and simple to implement.

- Ensure everything in the house works well: check electrics and plumbing; replace broken light bulbs and cracked window panes; make sure doors and windows don't stick. The fabric and mechanics of your home correspond to your body; keep them running smoothly and you should stay fit.
- Keep shapes soft and rounded where possible. Avoid sharp corners. Softly rounded sofas and chairs; big, squashy bean bags; and organic shapes are feng shui heaven.
- Boost the qi of your home by adding healthy green plants, fresh flowers and maybe a goldfish tank or water fountain.
- Hang wind chimes by your front door so they tinkle as you enter (they boost the energy of your home), but make sure they do not actually touch the door.
- Use mirrors to reflect pleasant views into the home. If you look out over an unpleasant view or a large building overshadows your home, hang a silver ball (from New Age stores) from a red ribbon in your window – this will deflect the harmful qi.
- Keep the toilet lid down! Otherwise, you will be simply flushing wealth energy away.

Vastu shastra

Vastu shastra is the Indian equivalent of feng shui, a complex science of spiritual architecture. In essence, the two systems are very similar. Both teach that, for good health, harmony and happiness we should live in symmetrical buildings and that there are beneficial directions in which to site the various rooms of the house and the furniture within it.

While feng shui has the *ba-gua*, a map of the various directions and the corresponding areas of life, vastu shastra has a mandala or sacred diagram called the vastu *purusha mandala*. The story goes that a formless being threatened to cause disruption between heaven and earth. The gods seized the creature and laid it face down on the earth, where it took the form of a human being (the *purusha*). Vastu practitioners say that the *mandala* (sacred image) forms the basis for understanding how energy moves through any given space.

Cosmic energy is said to enter a building through the *purusha*'s head in the northeast, move along its arms in the southeast and northwest, and finally gather at its feet in the southwest. So, to attract vital energy inside the home, it is crucial to keep the east, northeast and north clear, open and unobstructed. Once the energy has entered the house, it is important to ground it. So, the ground in the south and west is traditionally kept slightly higher and it has fewer openings, less open space and more solid walls.

Houses built according to vastu shastra principles generally face east to maximize the amount of early sunlight entering. In ancient India, the rising sun with its gentle heat and light was seen as a source of vitality, while the setting sun had far too much heat and glare. Ideally, every house and building should echo the sacred geometry of the cosmos, harnessing spiritual power and vital energy. This is spiritual architecture in its purest form – a kind of yoga for houses. So what do you do if your house doesn't face east or if your kitchen is in the wrong area? First and foremost, you should try to shift the rooms, so a vastu consultant may suggest you relocate your kitchen. Hardly a cheap option! However, there are more practicable ways to get round the problem. You may be advised that the cooker (stove) – the symbolic heart of the kitchen – be put in the south-east corner of the west room.

Although vastu shastra is complex, its practitioners promise it is well worth the effort. Applying vastu shastra to your home, they say, can bring you good health, great relationships, a happy family life and serious wealth.

Tips for vastu shastra success

GENERAL CONCEPTS
1 Houses should ideally be square or rectangular in shape – and sited within a square or rectangular plot of land. Avoid triangular or irregular plots.
2 The back of the house should be slightly higher than the front to contain the energy coming in the front door.
3 The front of your house should have more openings (doors and windows) than the back.
4 Ideally, your home should face east, to attract the energy of the sunrise. If it faces in another direction, ensure that east is kept open and is not blocked by trees or other buildings.
5 Never have three doors in a line – a very bad design in vastu shastra practice.
6 Avoid having your toilet in the northeast which is considered far from ideal.
7 The central part of the house is very sensitive. Do not have a staircase or a toilet here. Traditionally, this area would have been an open courtyard (impractical for most of us today), but do try to keep this area as clear, clean and stable as possible.

FRONT ENTRANCE AND HALL
1 Your front door should ideally face east. It should be the biggest door in the house.
2 Paint an 'ohm' symbol on your front door – at eye level – to improve your home's energy and vitality.
3 Always keep the area near the front door unobstructed and open, to allow the maximum amount of energy to flow into the house.
4 Place lower, lighter furniture near and around the front door. Any taller, heavier furniture should be placed in the area diagonally opposite (furthest away from the door) to hold the energy down.

BEDROOMS
1 The main bedroom should be in the southwest corner of the house or apartment. You should then sleep in the southwest corner of the room with your head facing south. If this is impossible, have your head facing west. It is not good to sleep with your head facing north.
2 Don't let your bed touch the walls on any side, as this will inhibit energy flow.
3 Children should sleep in the west corner of the house. Cots and beds should be in the southwest of the room so their heads face west. A green bulb will help enhance intelligence.

KITCHEN

1 If possible, place your kitchen in the southeast of the house – this is linked with the fire element in Vedic texts. Face the east when cooking. The sink should be towards the east of northeast.

2 To stimulate your appetite and that of your family, paint the walls soft pink or orange.

3 Place a mirror on the eastern wall to help strengthen your finances – good food mirrors financial strength.

DINING ROOM

1 The dining room should be a relaxed spot in which you can enjoy calm eating. Paint the walls soft pink, orange or cream.

2 Place a mirror on the east or north wall of your dining room, or perhaps even both.

3 Your dining table should be rectangular – avoid egg-shaped or irregular-shaped tables. Keep the dining table away from the walls of the room.

4 If possible, the dining room should be situated in the west of the house.

5 Paintings of the rising sun and the beauty of nature (without animals in them) will create a good feeling.

LIVING ROOM

1 Ideally, living rooms should be sited in the north, east or northeast part of the house.

2 Place furniture in the south and west, allowing plenty of space in the north and east of the room.

3 Put an indoor plant in a heavy pot in the south or west of the living room.

4 Recommended colours to use in your living room are white, soft blue and soft green.

5 Bless your living room to help attract beneficial energies to your home. Use incense, smudging (see page 98–9), clapping, drums, bells, prayer – whatever feels right for you.

Note: Feng shui and vastu shastra share many characteristics, but there are discrepancies between the two. The best advice is to follow the system to which you are intuitively drawn.

7 Relationships

Relationships can often seem like the greatest mystery of life. There are some people with whom we just 'click' – we feel as if we have been best friends all our lives. For others, we feel an instant attraction, an internal chemistry. Yet others seem to rub us the wrong way – almost before they speak or act. Psychologists hypothesize that we all have 'maps' that hardwire us to find some people more attractive than others, based on early experiences and family background. Astrologers attribute it to our star signs and those of the people we meet.

Whatever the reasons, there is no doubt that relationships can cause the greatest joy – and the greatest heartbreak – of all aspects of life. Most people would say that a good primary relationship is the most essential aspect of life, swiftly followed by close ties to family and friends. In this section, we're going to look at ways to improve our relationships.

The vital questions

If you want to check your relationship is on track, ask each other and yourself the following questions, devised by psychotherapists to gauge how well relationships are faring. They will help to pinpoint areas of potential difficulty and bring them out in the open for healthy discussion.

Decide whether you agree or disagree with each statement, and the level to which you agree or disagree.

1 I am happy with what my partner expects of me.
2 I agree with my partner's goals and plans.
3 I am satisfied with the ways in which we resolve our differences.
4 My partner is not too busy for us to do enough things together.
5 I am comfortable with my partner's different moods.
6 We agree on whether to have children, and how to raise them.
7 At times I need my personal space and my partner gives it to me.
8 I am happy with the way we show affection for each other.
9 I am not worried about being unsatisfied with my partner sexually.
10 We are able, when necessary, to talk out problems when we disagree.

Use your answers as the starting point for discussion with your partner. If you find it hard to understand your partner's point of view, try the empty-chair technique on page 26.

Keeping relationships on track

A good relationship needs careful nurturing, regular care and attention. It's not enough to cross your fingers and trust to luck that your partnership will flourish over the years – like a car, successful relationships need frequent servicing and regular check-ups. If your relationship is to run at peak performance, it needs regular maintenance. For healthy, happy relationships, some things need checking every day, some every week, while each month and year call for an in-depth overhaul. Try to insert the following into your emotional life.

Every day

- **SHARE YOUR WORRIES** We all lead tough, frantic lives. Many of us wage a constant struggle to balance work, children, household, friends, money, health. It's all too easy to find yourself wallowing in a pit of self-pity and forget that your partner has a tough life, too. Your relationship should be something that helps you both through the morass, not a further millstone round your neck. Try thinking about what would make his or her life better and, with a little luck, he or she will do the same for you. When you've had a tough day and you can't wait to unburden all your fury and frustration, wait – just 2 minutes – before you hurl it at your partner. Give each other a few minutes to enjoy just being in each other's company. Have a hug, hang on tight and appreciate that here's someone nice after all the monsters at work/on the bus/on the roads … and then, only then, should you launch into the 2-hour tirade against the world.
- **START THE DAY WITH A KISS** The alarm clock rings and you both stumble out of bed, in the perennial morning frenzy. Try setting the alarm for 5 minutes earlier and start your day with a kiss and a cuddle. Even if you are miles apart, you could always give each other a daily 'alarm call'. It only takes two minutes and starts the day on a happy note.
- **THINK ABOUT WHAT YOUR PARTNER WOULD LIKE** What would make his or her day? It doesn't have to be red roses or expensive presents, but how about taking his car through the carwash or buying him a bottle of his favourite Belgian beer, or putting on her favourite record? The most valued presents are often the most offbeat or the most simple: how about a birdfeeder for outside her office window; a subscription to the magazine she loves; a long, luxurious neck rub; or a ready-run bath with bubbles, candles and a glass of wine on the side?
- **MAKE TIME** Sometimes it's hard to remember you even live together, you see so little of each other. How about getting up just a little earlier to share breakfast, or even just coffee? Or a phone call at lunchtime? A good rule of thumb is to set aside 15–20 minutes to talk every day in order to debrief, catch up and say hello.
- **DON'T GO TO SLEEP ON AN ARGUMENT** Whatever it takes, try to stick to an agreement that you clear up anything that has annoyed you throughout the day before you turn off the light. That way you can start each day fresh.

Once a week

- **HAVE A SPECIAL NIGHT** Pick your least favourite day of the week. You could go to the cinema, for a walk in the country or out to eat. Or order in food and stay home with a video. Make time to give each other a massage or just talk.

- **CHECK OUT HOW YOU BOTH FEEL** Spend time each week finding out exactly how the other is feeling, voicing anxieties and irritations, and letting go of resentment, fear or anger. Pick a time when you aren't rushed. Maybe sit down with a glass of wine or have lunch together.
- **GIVE SMALL SURPRISES** Leave a note on the pillow when you have to get up before your partner does, or in the suitcase or underwear drawer if either one of you has to go away for a few days. Attach a simple note saying 'I love you' to a posy of flowers on the pillow, or a bar of sandalwood soap in the bathroom.
- **SET ASIDE TIME FOR SEX** We'll look more at this in the next section of the book, but, for now, use your imagination and experiment by changing your lovemaking scenario from time to time. For instance, you might want to break away from the mistaken idea that making love should only be done at night and in bed.

Once a month

- **SHARE AN ADVENTURE** Widen your horizons and do something completely different. Try something wild like hang gliding, horse riding or jet skiing. Take a weekend course in, say, massage, gourmet cookery or orienteering. You could spend a day at the races, an afternoon messing around in a rowing boat or take a picnic in the park. If you both fancy different things, make a list and take it in turns each month to try 'your' adventure.
- **HAVE AN ADVENTURE** – on your own. Every psychologist and relationship expert agrees we all need time out, time alone to pursue our own thoughts and interests, to see our own friends. Take time out to indulge yourself: a weekend in the country, a day's pampering at a health spa, an afternoon wandering round an art gallery or a long, self-indulgent lunch. Allow yourself some space and time. Absence really does make the heart grow fonder.
- **CHEERFULLY COMPROMISE** Once in a while, give him or her a special treat day. Choose all the things you know he or she loves: pottering around secondhand bookstores, watching football or trawling country pubs, a day's shopping, a smart lunch, perhaps a mini-facial and a soppy film. Just make sure you remember to have your special day, too.

Once a year

- **ASSESS YOUR RELATIONSHIP** Set aside time at least once a year to evaluate where you are as a couple. Ask yourselves questions. What values do we share? What do we both want right now? What do we both want for the future? Look at the current reality. What's working? What isn't? What do you appreciate or value about each other? How well does the relationship meet your needs? Look at possibilities. If the relationship could be any way you wanted it to be, how would it be? What would be different from the way things are now? Take your time. Set aside an evening (you could make it more appealing by including a nice dinner with wine and candles). Both of you should write down your answers to the questions above and then discuss them together – you might be surprised by the answers.
- **LEARN SOMETHING NEW** – together. Taking up horse riding or squash, chess or backgammon gives you a reason to spend regular time together and gives you new interests. Learn a language. When you're fluent, reward yourselves with a holiday to the country in question.

- **FANTASIZE** Write out a list of 100 things you each want to do in your life – from the mundane (have a haircut), through the interesting (learn ballroom dancing or raise ducks), to the extreme (travel round the world for a couple of years, change jobs or move to the country). Read out your lists and compare your wishes. You may well find fantasies in common – work towards turning them into reality. A shared goal can really cement a relationship.
- **MAKE A LONG-TERM COMMITMENT** If you aren't already married or living together, you don't necessarily have to go for an engagement ring or a house, but, if you are committed to your relationship, it helps to make a symbolic gesture. Anything could do: buy a washing machine together, rescue a dog from an animal refuge, take out a joint membership to the gym, or set up a joint savings account for the holiday of a lifetime. There is something powerful about seeing your names linked on an official document!
- **MAKE RITUALS** Set aside time once a year to celebrate your relationship – it's a way of spiritually rejuvenating your relationship. See more about rituals in Chapter 16. It doesn't have to be a strictly spiritual ritual: it might be treating yourselves to a smart hotel for a night or a break to Paris or Barcelona, or even a champagne breakfast in a hot-air balloon. You could incorporate some of the other ideas given here, such as listing your fantasies or checking out how you both feel about the relationship. Or you could just devote the time to sheer fun and enjoyment.

8 Sexuality

Touch is essential for both our physical and our psychological health. Research has even shown that premature babies need touch in order to grow normally. We certainly don't lose that need for closeness, warmth and touch as we get older – touch is also life-sustaining for us as adults. And there is nothing so close, so intimate and so totally accepting as the touch of one lover on another. Sex makes us feel more than just desirable – it allows us to feel wanted, cared for, protected and safe. It makes us feel good about ourselves.

Why sex is good for you

A good sex life is incredibly beneficial for our health and wellbeing. Here's why.
- **IT REDUCES STRESS** Sex releases chemicals in much the same way as intense physical exercise does. In addition, during lovemaking, the muscles of the body become highly tensed; following orgasm, the body completely relaxes. Sex is like a very extreme version of the relaxation exercise known as progressive relaxation, where you move through the body tensing and then relaxing each set of muscles. During sex, however, your body does this automatically and to a much greater degree. A large study by the Institute for Advanced Study of Human Sexuality confirms the theory that people who have fulfilling and happy sex lives generally show far fewer stress symptoms than those who don't: they are less anxious, less violent and hostile, and are far less likely to blame their misfortunes on others.
- **IT MAKES US FEEL BETTER ABOUT OURSELVES** A healthy, happy sex life can boost our self-esteem like nothing on earth. No other activity is so intimate, so personal – it's like baring your very soul. When your partner responds with love and affection, it bestows a sense of wholeness. Of course, sex will only boost your self-esteem if you're with the right partner.
- **IT SOOTHES SLEEPLESSNESS** A bout of lovemaking is probably the last thing you would think of when you can't get to sleep. Yet research shows that an orgasm can be the perfect trigger to a good night's sleep because serotonin (the hormone that induces sleepiness) is released after orgasm. Also, insomnia is most often brought on by anxiety and tension. Sex relieves that tension.
- **IT CAN HELP TO HEAL SORROW AND GRIEF** Expressing ourselves through sex can have a profound healing effect. When you're feeling depressed or sad, it's all too easy to withdraw into yourself. Lovemaking makes you connect with another person at a very deep, nurturing level. Sex also produces endorphins, feelgood hormones that elevate mood, so a session of sex when you're feeling low could be the best possible antidepressant.

- **IT HEALS YOUR HEART** Sex really can provide you with a mini-workout (it's been estimated that a woman burns around 4.2 calories a minute during sex, compared to 4 calories per minute playing tennis). Obviously, you're not going to keep going long enough to notch up as many calories as a full tennis match, but you will still give a toning effect to your heart and lungs. However, sex also has far more subtle effects on the health of our hearts. A prime risk factor for heart disease is lack of love. One study looked at the sex lives of women hospitalized for heart attacks. Of these, 65 per cent reported some form of sexual dissatisfaction or frigidity. For a control group, the researchers asked the same questions of women hospitalized for non-heart-related problems and only 24 per cent said they had difficult or non-existent sex lives.
- **IT COULD EXTEND YOUR LIFE** There appears to be a strong connection between immunity and sex – a healthy sex life can make us more resistant to disease and stress. It seems that the arousal, excitement and physical release of sexual activity enhances the natural ability of the immune system to ward off illness. A typical orgasm boosts the body's T3 and T4 lymphocyte cells (the ones that fight infection) by up to 20 per cent. This comes as no surprise to many alternative practitioners, who have long believed that touch alone can help improve immune function. A study at the University of Miami seems to prove the point: massage alone raises levels of serotonin, the neurotransmitter that triggers the increase of immune-defence cells.

How to use sexual energy to help and heal

In order to have health-giving sex, you need to have a healthy, open, honest relationship. Here's how to pave the way ...

- Make sure you both really enjoy your lovemaking. The art of a truly happy sex life is good communication, say sex therapists and relationship experts. Talk about sex – about what you enjoy and what you don't like as much. Be honest, but careful – don't blame your partner, just say how you feel.
- Become sensual as well as sexual in your everyday life. Give your body and mind sensual treats: this means eating and exercising well; wearing clothing that feels good on your skin; enjoying a languid bath with essential oils, or an invigorating shower. Engage your senses to the full.
- Learn how to give a simple massage and have your partner learn, too. There are plenty of books and videos giving simple instructions, or follow the instructions on page 53.
- If you seem never to have time for lovemaking, make a regular 'appointment' for sex. Although it may sound rather unromantic, sex therapists all agree that these appointments can do wonders for your sex life – adding a frisson of anticipation to the day.
- Give yourselves enough time. The most frequent reason for women being dissatisfied with sex is that they feel they are not given enough time and attention. Lovemaking is a vital part of your relationship: allow it the time it deserves.
- Keep the romance alive in your life: give your partner small surprises. This need not mean flowers. It could be a new book or CD; a photo frame with a picture of you in it; or a favourite food or drink. Leave a loving message – on the bed, on the answerphone, on e-mail. Suggest a surprise outing or have a picnic in bed. Revitalize your love life with books and videos. Bring a new element into your bedroom with fresh ideas: books such as Anne Hooper's *Kama Sutra* (Dorling Kindersley) make for fun bedtime reading. If you are interested in Tantra (where sex meets mysticism), read the books by Margo Anand (*The Art of Sexual Ecstasy* and *The Art of Sexual Magic*, both Piatkus).

- Turn your bedroom into a private sanctuary. Avoid having work in the bedroom, take out the television, put a lock on the door so you know you can have privacy. Make it really comfortable – add sumptuous velvet cushions (according to feng shui, they should be red or deep pink).

The art of sacred sex

The ancient Indian art of Tantrism teaches union with God through lovemaking. In the original tradition, sex was merely a means to an end: adepts were not seeking better orgasms, but a deeper religious experience. Here in the West, few of us are prepared to complete the years of arduous training that a Tantric has to undergo. However, practising aspects of Tantrism can have a remarkable effect on your love life – and on your relationship with your partner. The ritual given here is based loosely on the complex Tantric ceremony known as *maithuna*. It can give surprisingly intense results very swiftly.

1 Make sure your bedroom is as beautiful and sensual as it can possibly be. Follow the guidelines already given above, paying attention to the look of the room, the scent of it, the sounds around you and the feel of coverings. Red candles can provide soft, sensual lighting and suggest passion.

2 Prepare a tray of delicious, exotic finger food (just small nibbles, not a heavy meal). Add a decanter of wine and two beautiful glasses (be careful not to overdo the wine).

3 Both of you should shower or bathe (either separately or together). Spend time connecting with your body. Dress in light, flowing clothes.

4 Sit down and spend time simply enjoying each other's company, talking, eating and drinking together. You may feel moved to touch and caress each other. You might want to try some yoga together or breathing in time with one another, or simply sit gazing deep into each other's eyes.

5 You may already feel aroused. To prepare yourselves for sacred intercourse, however, the man should meditate on the image of the vulva, the yoni, picturing it as warm, welcoming, moist and soft, opening and closing like a flower. Concentrate on the soft aroma of musk and imagine the sound of a deep heartbeat, a slow rhythm of the earth, the pulse of life.

6 The woman, meanwhile, meditates on the penis, the lingam, visualizing it as erect, mentally examining its different textures. The scent to imagine is patchouli. The sound is that of a faster, more insistent throb.

7 The man should now move gently forwards and enter the woman deeply and solidly. Any position can be adopted, but many people prefer sitting face to face.

8 For a while just move slowly, the woman milking the penis (squeezing and releasing it with her vaginal muscles) and the man thrusting gently.

9 Next, allow yourselves to become totally still. Stare deeply into each other's eyes. Imagine yourselves linked at the various chakras: at the head, the throat, the heart, the solar plexus and particularly the genitals.

10 Imagine your entire genital area surrounded by a pulsing orb of deep red light.

11 Now synchronize your breathing, slowly and deeply breathing towards your partner's mouth.

12 Imagine the energy generated from your genitals spreading up your spines and throughout your entire bodies. Remain in this position for as long as is comfortable. Even if you manage just a few minutes, it should still result in an unusual experience for you and your partner.

Sensual massage

Giving and receiving massage is a wonderful way to relax and to foster love and trust. It helps you both become aware of each other's bodies in a safe, loving way. It is also deeply sensual and the perfect prelude to lovemaking. Don't worry that the massage won't be perfect or professional enough. The aim is to give your partner pleasure, and almost any touch (providing it feels good to your partner) will do that.

1 Make your bedroom comfortable and pleasant. Make sure it is warm enough, clear the clutter and (because oils may stain) put a towel over the bed or wherever you intend to give the massage. Choose some relaxing music you both like. You may want to light some candles and burn some relaxing essential oils (lavender or camomile) or romantic oils (such as sandalwood or ylang ylang) in a burner.

2 Make up your massage oil. Use 8 drops of one of the oils above in 4 teaspoons of a base oil such as sweet almond.

3 Start on the back with your thumbs on either side of the spine, fingers pointing towards the neck. Allow your hands to glide slowly up the body and around the shoulders. Draw your hands lightly down the side of the back to your starting position. Don't worry if your technique is a bit stilted to begin with – just relax and ask your partner for feedback (he or she might like your touch to be firmer, or gentler).

4 Fleshy areas such as hips and thighs can be kneaded gently. Lift, squeeze and roll the skin between the thumb and fingers of one hand and glide it towards the other hand.

5 Curl your fingers into loose fists, keeping the fingers (not the knuckles) against the skin. Work all over the body. Make small circling movements on the shoulders, palms of the hands, soles of the feet and chest.

6 Form your hands into cup shapes and, with quick, light movements, move over the skin as if beating a drum.

7 If you feel adventurous, emulate Hawaiian masseurs, who use their entire arms or their hair to touch the body.

8 Gauge how your partner feels (if you can't tell, ask!). If they are in the mood for sex, kiss them gently all over. Very softly stroke the thighs and breasts, gradually moving into lovemaking.

9 Family

We all want to play happy families. We'd all like to be calm, gentle, wise grown-ups who have perfect relationships with our loving partners and our happy, confident children. Unfortunately, most families end up bickering and squabbling, sulking and screaming at some point. How can you talk to a child who simply doesn't want to listen? How can you give your partner, your children and yourself the time you all need? How can you protect your family from the dangers within the society in which we live? Happy families is certainly no game; it's more like mission impossible.

When you stop to think about it, it's not that surprising. These are the people with whom we live intimately; the people who see our bad sides as well as our good; the ones who have to put up with our horrible habits, our lousy moods, our everyday frustrations and irritations. It is simply not reasonable or realistic to expect to have the 'perfect' family all the time. There are plenty of things you can do, however, to make your home a happier place and to bring more joy and fewer frayed tempers to family relationships.

Ways to promote peace

- **LISTEN** Often misunderstandings arise because we simply don't listen to each other. Children feel hurt and ignored. Partners feel left out. Make time to listen.
- **PRESS THE PAUSE BUTTON** Everyone needs a remote control with 'pause' on it, to be used before we lash out at the people around us. It's natural to want to hit back when someone hurts us, but resist the urge. Think how your reaction will affect the other person before you reply.
- **BE NICE** That's a tough one, isn't it? Bring the principle of 'random acts of kindness' into family life. Think of little things that make people's lives easier or more pleasant. It could be taping a favourite television programme if someone's out; it may be doing the washing up; it may be cooking a favourite meal or picking a posy of wild flowers.
- **STOP NAGGING** Resist the urge to criticize and complain: give each other compliments, rather than constant nagging. Think of something nice to say to everyone regularly. When you're wrong, apologize. We all make mistakes, so say sorry and mean it. Hard as it may be, don't nag children all the time: let go of the little things and boost their confidence by letting them 'win' sometimes. Toddlers going through the 'no' stage can be particularly testing. Make a few totally rigid rules (about consideration and safety) and let the unimportant things go.

- **BE LOYAL AND RELIABLE** Keep any promises you make – always. Be loyal at all times to your family. Defend its members when they're not around. Let go of grudges. Yes, we all make mistakes, we all do rotten things from time to time, but try not to hold on to grudges for hours, weeks, months or even years! Let go of the past and start afresh.
- **SPEND TIME TOGETHER** Set aside certain times during the week when you act together as a family. Perhaps you can make it Sunday lunch or an evening when you all go out (for a walk, to the movies). Let everyone have an input – take it in turns to choose what the outing will be.

Your family space

When we live alone, we can organize your space exactly as we want it. Once we start sharing our homes with a family, however, the issue of personal space really comes to the fore. We all have varying requirements and a home needs to reflect everyone's wishes and desires. Not paying attention to this oft-forgotten aspect of family life can be the source of a lot of grudges and unhappiness. Spend some time on this exercise.

1 First, you need to draw a floor plan of your home. It need not be draughtsman quality, but try to make the proportions roughly accurate. If your home has several floors, do a plan for each one. Make several copies and let everyone in the house have their own to colour.
2 Label each room on your plan and mark in all the major pieces of furniture.
3 Pick a colour for each family member and start to colour in the plan. Think about who uses each space and mark it accordingly (you may have stripes in some places!). For example, someone may have a chair that is supremely 'theirs'.
4 Let the colours show the division of tasks in the house. One person may do all the cooking, so the cooker (stove) is 'theirs', or even the whole kitchen – bar the table where you eat! The table may be commandeered for homework by the children, however, and so be shared.
5 Balance out how much each person uses each room and colour in the room accordingly.

What you end up with may well prove surprising. You may have colonized huge parts of the house for yourself or you may realize that you have been virtually squeezed out. The children may have no place to call their own. Certain rooms may be out of bounds to certain people. Have a good, long think about why this might be – and if it really suits your needs.

Of course, different people in the family may have different perceptions of how the space is used. View the plans as providing a starting point for a debate, and try to be fair.

- Is the division of space fair?
- Who wants or needs more?
- Can you think, together, of ways that would give everyone what he or she needs?

This may seem impossible, but a solution can usually be found. For example, some people need certain spaces only at particular times. It could be perfectly fine for the kitchen to be a homework zone, providing the books are cleared away afterwards so an adult can use the space for making pottery or writing the great novel! Children sharing a bedroom need to have their 'own' walls for posters and such, or they could divide the space with furniture or a decorative screen.

What kind of family do you want?

Few of us stop to think about what we actually want from our families. Often we express our thoughts only in negative terms: we don't want a family like the one we grew up in or we don't want to be like so-and-so ... Change the focus and think what you do want.

Set aside an evening to discuss your 'ideal' family, your goals and aspirations – what you see as your 'purpose' as a family. It could be a nice idea to have a special family meal beforehand and then discuss the following.

- What kind of family do you really want to be? What words come to mind when you think about your ideal family?
- To what kind of home would you like to invite your friends?
- What embarrasses you about your family? Don't be nasty or vindictive, but do be honest.
- What do you love about your family? What makes you feel warm and good? What makes you want to come home? If your feelings about family and home are negative, is there anything that feels good about it?
- If you had to write a 'mission statement' for your family for the coming year, what would it be?

Sit down and talk about this. Above all, listen – every family member should have a say. You might be surprised by what is important to each of you. This could provide the basis for an important family heart-to-heart. Together, come up with a short list of the things that are most important to you all about your family. You may wish to write them up on a large card or poster, which could be put somewhere you can all see it and act as a reminder of what your family is about.

10 Dreamworking

Dreams are the medium through which our unconscious minds try to communicate with us. Most of us, however, ignore these messages from the night. This is a shame, as our conscious minds are so overloaded with all the practical considerations, fears and conventions of everyday life that we often cannot see the wood for the trees. Our unconscious, free of such restrictions, generally knows precisely what we really need. Learn to listen to your unconscious and it could help make your waking life much more fulfilling. Your relationships should improve, your career could change – listening to your unconscious could even help your health.

We spend a third of our lives asleep and, even though you may not remember your dreams, there is no doubt that we all, without exception, dream each and every night. It's curious, therefore that so few people bother to consult the oracle in their own heads. The concept of dreamworking is nothing new. The Old Testament is full of references to prophetic dreams, while in ancient Greece people would regularly spend a therapeutic night in a Temple of Sleep, where they believed the god of the temple would send healing dreams. Native Americans have used the power of dreaming for centuries – they would regard ignoring a dream as sheer stupidity.

In the West, however, dreaming has been very much marginalized for centuries, dismissed as either florid imagination or simply the mind's way of disposing of the detritus of the day. It wasn't until Sigmund Freud started investigating dreams that these pyrotechnics of the night started to be taken seriously. Yet even Freud saw dreams simply as repositories for all that lies repressed in human nature. It was left to Carl Jung to map the dream world and it is Jung that most modern dream therapists follow when they travel into the land of night.

Working with your dreams can equip you with a passport to a renewed sense of creativity. It can be a fresh way of tackling tricky problems and relationships. Our dreams can offer us a means of realizing our deepest desires and coming to terms with our deepest fears.

Dreams can often suggest solutions of which the waking mind has not the faintest glimmer. One woman suffered a humiliating harangue from her boss at work. That night, she dreamed of her hated school headmistress and was struck by the comparison between the two authority figures. She realized that she was feeling exactly the same sense of power-lessness, helplessness and childlike desire for revenge that she had felt as a child. The perception made her snap out of this childish response and remain level-headed.

Working even more deeply, dreams offer us a direct route to the past. They give us a second chance, an opportunity to look back at our mistakes, traumas and hurts, and reassess them in the bright light of the present. Many psychotherapists of various dis-ciplines will use dreamwork in this way, unravelling the past and often, in the process, leading their clients to a far greater sense of perspective and of ease. Interestingly, it is not only emotional or mental relief that comes from working with the past. Often, physical symptoms will disappear when you uncover the original reason for becoming tense or stiff. This experience can be powerful and sometimes painful; many people may feel more comfortable working with a trained therapist for this aspect of dreamwork.

However, you can still go a long way on your own, if you are prepared to be totally honest about the past. All too often we tend to see what we want to see, to discover what we want to discover. It could be a good idea to enlist the help of a close friend, who could perhaps point out an interpretation we might avoid ourselves (although, ultimately, it is your dream and only you can say what it really means).

Above all, don't deny your dreams. Even if they appear disturbing, distressing or even disgusting, they might have a purpose. A little time spent working out their messages, trying to understand the meaning behind their symbols, could make your waking life far easier and more pleasant. In other words, make friends with them – however seemingly mad or bad. Like all good friends, they will in return do their best to help and support you.

Recalling your dreams

Before you can even start to work with your dreams, you have to be able to recall them in the first place. There is no one, infallible way to remember dreams. Some people find that simply saying aloud before sleep that they want to remember their dreams helps. Some ask for a dream on a particular topic. Others meditate. Still others just wait to see what happens. There are, however, a few points which seem to be of universal help:

- On waking, it can help to stay lying still in your sleeping body position to recall your dream.
- Try saying it aloud or telling someone else your dream as soon as you wake.
- Having a 'dream book' or journal by your bed to write in as soon as you open your eyes can be a very useful way of capturing a dream. Sometimes writing down and rereading your dreams can aid in understanding them. If you prefer, draw an image that sums up your dream.
- Sometimes a simple ritual before sleep, such as spending 10 minutes gazing at a candle or into a glass of water, burning aromatic herbs or dancing to a favourite piece of music, can help lead us into dreams.

Exploring dreams, talking to your dreams

How can you work with your dreams once you have recalled them? Try these simple techniques.

- Say you dream of the sea, a lion or a school. Don't race to find a dream dictionary and simply look up the symbol. It isn't as straightforward as that. You need to think about the personal associations you may have with the sea or with a lion. Write down everything of which it reminds you. Often quite surprising insights can appear and frequently the symbol will draw into your conscious mind long-forgotten incidents from the past.
- Use the empty-chair technique (see page 26). Take two chairs or two cushions. Sit yourself on one and imagine your dream (or a figure from it) is sitting on the other.

Try speaking to your dreams, telling them how much you want to remember them. You may feel silly at first, but persevere, as it can be very illuminating. Switch seats and speak as if you were the dream replying. Say whatever comes into your mind, without censoring it or feeling embarrassed. Give the dream a voice – let it describe itself and tell you what would help it to surface. You may well be very surprised at what comes up.

- A creative way to start exploring dreams is through painting or drawing them (see the section on art therapy on pages 65–6). The result may be a literal picture of what happened in the dream or it may be more of an expression of the mood of the dream through shape and colour. Don't ask other people to 'interpret' your painting, although it can be helpful to discuss it with someone else. Ask them what they notice about it.
- Use the technique of 'dreaming your dream on', otherwise known as 'active imagination'. If a dream finishes on an uncertain or disconcerting note, try continuing it in waking time. To get in the right frame of mind, find a quiet, dark place where you won't be disturbed and let yourself deeply relax. Start to imagine your dream in all its detail, not just visually, but with all your senses – hearing the sounds, accessing the feeling in your body. There may be a vivid character in the dream whom you want to question. If so, simply ask the character if it would like to talk to you and then wait for the answer. Be patient: you have to wait for the reply and not rush to give it yourself. You will get a sense of when it's coming and, in this way, it won't just be something your conscious mind is making up.

Who do you meet in your dreams?

Generally, the people whom you meet in dreams will tend to be different aspects of yourself, often those repressed in waking life. There are no hard and fast rules – and it isn't worth looking up your figure in a 'dream dictionary' – but these are some common correspondences.

- **THE SHADOW** One powerful image that often appears is the 'shadow', a dream character that normally manifests as someone of the same sex as yourself. Jung said that the shadow represents all the things about ourselves which we find unacceptable and so try to repress. Hence, if expressing or feeling anger wasn't acceptable in your family as you grew up, your shadow may appear as an angry or violent man or woman. If you can talk to your shadow and become on good terms, it will allow you to express your anger appropriately without flying off the handle. Ruthlessness is a common shadow for women because lots of little girls aren't allowed to be ruthless. Try putting your shadow in the 'other' chair in the empty-chair technique (see above).
- **THE QUEEN** A very common image in dreams is the queen, which, for a woman, usually represents her sovereignty and power. For a man, the queen tends to represent his ability to deal with the feminine side of his nature.
- **ROCKS STARS AND FILM STARS** These generally represent the hero, excitement and creativity. Dreaming about a star means you want to project the part of you that craves attention and the centre stage.
- **BABIES** These represent new life of all kinds. Dreaming of babies often occurs when people need to develop other sides of themselves – often when their children have grown up and left home.

Unpleasant dreams

Don't be disgusted or horrified by your dreams – no matter how vile they may appear to your waking, conscious self. There are messages in every dream, however disturbing.

- **GOING TO THE TOILET IN PUBLIC** This is a very common dream. Urinating in public usually represents spontaneous self-expression, while defecating generally represents your creativity. Either of these dreams usually means you haven't yet found your true way of expressing yourself.
- **BEING NAKED IN THE STREET** Another common albeit disconcerting dream, this classically indicates a fear of revealing who you really are. Normally, it will suggest that you need to reveal more of your true personality.
- **BEING CHASED** Usually, whatever or whomever is chasing you represents an aspect of yourself that wants to make contact with you. Animals can represent your instinctual nature – it may be that you are leading too cerebral a life. Try talking to the creature or using the empty-chair technique (see pages 58–9).
- **HAVING SEX** Jung found that sexual dreams usually signify creativity. If you are making love with someone of the same sex as yourself, this usually indicates that you are trying to get in touch with your own feminine or masculine energy.
- **TAKING EXAMS** A common dream in which you realize that you are due to take an exam (or speak in public or run a race, etc.) yet have not done the necessary preparation. This indicates anxiety and fears that may be holding you back. Maybe you're a perfectionist with unrealistic expectations of yourself – try to be less critical.

11 Creativity

When we were young, we probably sang at the tops of our voices; we twirled and danced, fancying ourselves ballerinas; we painted and drew without giving a thought to whether the result was 'Art' (with a capital 'A') or not. As we grow older, however, we tend to give up artistic pursuits and leave them to children or the professionals. Yes, we may venture onto the dance floor (providing we've had a few drinks for Dutch courage), we may even sing along with the radio (providing no one's listening), but that's about it.

A growing band of therapists are claiming, however, that if we could only get back to that childlike enjoyment of art, dance and song, we could all become much healthier and happier. Over the next few pages, we'll take a look at simple ways to kickstart your creativity.

Dance therapy

All forms of dance are wonderful self-therapy. Dancing is one of the primal instincts of humankind: from the dawn of time, we have felt the urge to move our bodies in a rhythmic way. In fact, dance was originally often a sacred urge – dance would bring the community together for celebration, for sacrifice and to mark the passing seasons of the year and the seasons of life. In our modern Western culture, we have lost touch with our dance heritage. We no longer dance to conjure up the deer for good hunting. (Why bother when our food is lying prepackaged on the supermarket counter?) We no longer dance to honour the earth; instead, we trample all over it. Yes, we dance at weddings and the odd Christmas party, but we no longer leap over the Beltane fires or spin around to welcome the rising energy of the new year. Yet, in losing our dance, we have lost part of our souls.

On the most basic level, dancing is good exercise – it gives your cardiovascular system a workout and stretches your muscles. It's also a wonderful form of stress relief. It really doesn't matter which kind of dance you choose. If you've always fancied floating around a ballroom, why not start now? If serene circle dancing seems suitable, join a circle (it's blissfully calming). If, on the other hand, you fancy kicking up a storm with salsa, Irish jigging or Ceroc, go for it. Of course, it need not be organized dance – you may feel able to connect with your inner self or the earth and start to move. Most of us, however, have lost the knack. That's why some forms of dance have been specifically designed to produce a deep therapeutic effect on mind and body. One of my favourites is Biodanza.

Biodanza

While most dancing leaves you totally exhausted, Biodanza leaves you bouncing with boundless energy. It can take away stress and improve your sleep; it can even give you the nerve to chuck no-good lovers and begin new relationships. After a year of Biodanza, its growing band of aficionados swear, your life will be totally different.

Biodanza is tricky to categorize: it's much more than a dance form, but it's not technically a therapy and Biodanza's practitioners certainly don't like to tout it as a cure. Its creator, Chilean psychologist and anthropologist Rolando Toro, came up with the idea for Biodanza back in 1960. He wanted to reintroduce a dance that could express deep feelings and allow people to really connect to each other. He felt that, by dancing in a manner true to our essential 'inner' self, we could literally dance ourselves back to health and happiness, learning to love our bodies and to feel happier in society. He worked at first with mentally disturbed patients and discovered that certain kinds of music would make them move in different ways. This would, in turn, bring about startling changes, in both their bodies and their emotions. Research showed that the moves were stimulating different parts of the nervous system.

The theory is quite complicated, but the dance itself is simple and great fun. Now well established in the USA, South America, Switzerland, Italy and France, Biodanza is used not just for general wellbeing, but also as a specific therapy for people with eating disorders, those with mental disabilities, children with autism or Down's syndrome, and people suffering from asthma, cardiovascular problems, Parkinson's disease, osteoporosis or gastrointestinal disorders. The very young, the very old, pregnant women – everyone can benefit.

There is absolutely no need to be a 'good' dancer. There is no 'correct' way of doing exercises. The point is to find your own dance. As Rolando Toro puts it: 'Our proposal is to dance to our own life. To retrieve the condition of being the owners of our body, our emotions, as a whole, a unit.'

Writing

Many of us dream of writing a novel, penning poems or scribbling an autobiography, yet few of us ever knuckle down to it. We find plenty of excuses – we don't have time, we were never 'good' at writing, nobody would want to read what we have to say. The words remain unwritten. That's a pity, because writing can act as a potent form of self-therapy, illuminating the past and helping us understand ourselves in the present. Writing freely can clear emotional blocks, unshackle creativity and help us in almost every area of life.

It's not about writing a bestseller – although, once the creative juices start flowing, you may end up a published author. It's more about freeing yourself from writing's taboos and learning how to access your innermost feelings.

Psychologists have long recommended we keep journals to record our daily thoughts, claiming that writing down our innermost thoughts and feelings, uncensored, can help emotional growth. Freud pioneered free-association (saying or writing whatever 'pops' into your head), while Jung advocated 'active imagination' (letting the imagination run free to explore dreams or fantasies). Let's look at some simple ways to use the written word as therapy – and for fun.

You will need to set aside a decent amount of time for these exercises – at least 10 minutes for the actual writing of each exercise, plus time to settle yourself beforehand and some time afterwards to muse on what happened in the exercise. Pick a time when and place where you won't be disturbed – you won't be able to write just what you feel if you know someone is going to pop up behind you and read over your shoulder! Choose a pen that feels comfortable and writes easily, and either loose sheets of paper or (if you intend to keep a record of your work) a bound notebook.

Before you start, it may be a good idea to sit quietly for a few minutes and focus on your breathing, allowing yourself to become calm. You may like to light a candle or burn some aromatherapy oil to give yourself a sense of ritual.

Get in touch with your feelings

Start by trying out different ways of writing about your feelings, thoughts and attitudes. It doesn't matter if what you write is absolute rubbish, embarrassing, fanciful or whatever. Nobody else need ever see it. Try these exercises – just for fun. Work quickly, so you don't have time to censor yourself.

1 **RIGHT HERE, RIGHT NOW** Start by looking at your immediate surroundings. What catches your attention? It could be your cat curled up on a sofa, the rain on the window panes, a cobweb in a corner. Describe two or three of the things you notice, being very precise in your descriptions: what do they look like, smell like, feel like, taste(!) like? How do they make you feel? What thoughts come into your head when you describe them? What is your mood, your feelings, your thoughts? Keep writing for about 12 minutes on this.

2 **A SPECIAL PLACE** We all have 'special' places of the past, most usually from childhood. What outside places do you remember from when you were small? It might be a beach, a playground, a small patch of land that was magical to you. Describe the place in as much detail as you can – again, think about using all your senses. How do you feel about this place now? How did you feel then? What happened in that place? Again, spend about 12 minutes on this exercise.

3 **DESERT ISLAND THOUGHTS** Imagine you are marooned on a desert island – it's beautiful and safe, with plenty of food and water, and a nice shelter. Think about the following:
   • What and whom would you most miss? Why?
   • What wouldn't you miss? Why?
   • Which three things would be your desert island objects (excluding things such as television, computer, telephone!)?
   • What would be your one desert island book?
   • How would you live from day to day? Would you be able to cope with being alone? How would you do it?

Flow-writing

This technique works at unleashing the huge reservoir of ideas, images and feelings that make up our unconscious minds. Our minds are like giant icebergs; only a tiny part (the conscious mind) appears above the water. Below lies a huge mass of unconscious (but highly important) information. Flow-writing bypasses the controlling conscious mind and allows this hidden material to come to the surface.

You will probably want desperately to direct your writing, but resist the urge. Don't plan, just write whatever comes into your head. Don't worry if you panic or dry up. Simply repeat the last few words you've written until something new suggests itself, then continue. Try not to censor yourself – it doesn't matter if what you write seems trivial or silly. Equally, it's fine if embarrassing or private feelings come up. This is for you — nobody else ever need read it. Don't worry about whether you have the right word or your writing is logical or your grammar perfect – just 'go with the flow'.

If you find this hard, start off with one of these sentences:

'For the first time in my life I ...'
'In my heart of hearts, I really wanted to ...'
'It's been many years since ...'
'My deepest fear was that ...'
'Nobody ever knew that ...'

After you have written each piece, underline any sentences, phrases and words that catch your attention. You may find that one of these phrases or words is the impetus for a fresh bout of flow-writing. You can use this technique if you know you have an area you want to explore. Simply pick a sentence that plugs you into that time or incident, and off you go.

Using sound for healing

You don't have to be a singer or have a good voice to benefit from singing, toning or making sounds. It isn't about perfect pitch or making a beautiful sound: it's all about gaining confidence and being who you want to be.

'So many people were told they couldn't sing at school,' says sound therapist Susan Lever, 'that they were tone deaf or maybe told off when they were singing and it stops them enjoying singing. We have a lot of early messages that it's not okay to be who we are. Sometimes we try to copy other people's voices, we try to get rid of dialects or we have "telephone voices". Playing with sound helps people feel safe. They can relax and feel it's okay to take risks and explore.'

First of all, take a look at the ideas on sound therapy (pages 77–9). Groaning, sighing and humming are simple, effective ways to start using your voice.

Take every opportunity you can to use your voice – sing along to the radio while you're doing the housework, belt out rock tunes or opera arias as you drive in your car. If you can find somewhere really private, you might even try screaming. Many therapists say that, if you can unleash your inner scream (and apparently most of us have one), you can plug into some deep, powerful feelings – and at the same time release a lot of stress and tension.

Making sound can really change your mood. If you feel low and you make happy sounds, it will lift you without a doubt. Your breathing will automatically change and so will your physiological state. You will find you have a lot more energy, a lot more confidence and a lot less stress.

Above all, the aim is to find your natural voice and relearn how to speak and sing without strain or effort. Often that involves relaxing and teaching yourself to let the voice come naturally from the whole body, rather than holding it tight in the throat. Once this happens, you may discover some surprising side effects. Letting your voice come from your whole body will often start to release long-standing blocks and tensions. If you *have* always spoken or sung from your throat, it is probably a protection mechanism. Start singing from your heart or your abdomen and you might find something else coming up, such as old grief, hurt or anger.

Art as therapy – painting your way to health

Daubing paint or scribbling with a pencil, say art therapists, has the power to heal. You don't have to be Van Gogh and you don't need any art-school techniques. Painting whatever you want to, straight from the heart, can apparently put you in touch with repressed emotions and long-buried hurts.

Psychologists explain that art has the ability to bypass our conscious, 'thinking' mind and connect directly with our subconscious, where all our deepest fears and hurts are buried. Paint and you could discover hidden sides to your personality; you could gain in confidence and self-esteem; you might even find that physical ailments disappear or are alleviated when you allow yourself a creative outlet.

Art has been used as a tool by psychotherapists since 1810. Since then, many experts have discovered that, when people paint freely, they are able to express feelings and give a form on paper to fears and terrors that they are utterly unable to express in words. Art therapy is most definitely not about painting or drawing 'properly': you don't have to make pretty or lifelike pictures, but rather simply pick up your paintbrush and see what happens. Art therapist Michael Edwards suggests you sit quietly and breathe deeply before painting. Then just see what appears on the paper. Afterwards, he suggests you try 'talking to your pictures'. It sounds crazy, but he promises that you could have some very interesting responses. 'Write a commentary or simply scribble a letter to your painting. Ask it questions: it might answer. I know it sounds nuts, but it does seem to work.'

The process isn't always easy or fun. Art leads people gently into their psyches. Sometimes distressing things come up, but somehow they can be contained by the paper. In other words, you might feel terrified about, say, a nightmare, but by painting it out you can take back a certain amount of control over your fears. Art therapists are loath to claim miracles, but sometimes people even find physical problems disappear.

Healing your mind and soul with art

To get a feel for art therapy, try these exercises. As with all these creative exercises, you should find a time when and a place where you won't be disturbed. It doesn't matter which art materials you choose – some people like to paint large (on huge sheets of paper or newspaper) with poster paints; others prefer scribbling on smaller sheets with felt pens, crayons, chalks or charcoal. You could go to an art shop and see which materials draw you. Don't censor your choice – one woman I met found she worked best painting on glass!

- Put aside all expectations of painting a 'proper' picture. That isn't the point. You may not even paint anything recognizable. Some people simply use colour or shapes or symbols. Others don't use paintbrushes – they prefer to splat paint on with their hands or fingers, or even feet!
- You may find it's easier to paint with your non-dominant hand (so, if you're left-handed, try using your right hand). Perhaps you could shut your eyes while you paint. Maybe you could even dance as you paint! All these suggestions tend to free your unconscious and allow it to take over.

Do-it-yourself art therapy

- **PAINT YOUR LIFELINE** Take a large piece of paper and any art materials you like. Imagine that the paper represents your lifetime – the beginning, the now, the future and the end. Sit quietly for a few moments and then fill the paper in whatever way you like. Don't expect anything or try to draw 'properly'; use whatever symbols or images you feel are appropriate. You might choose to depict events in your life or simply choose different colours to represent different parts of your life or feelings. When you have finished, be aware of how you feel – both in your mind and your body. What is your painting saying? Does it yield clues to how you think or how you feel about your life? What are the themes and questions in it? Don't throw it away afterwards – keep it and look at it from time to time to see if any new insights arise.

- **PAINT A FAIRY STORY** Fairy tales and myths have powerful effects on our psyches. Think back to your childhood – is there one particular story you remember? It may be a favourite or one that frightened you at the time. If you don't have a particular tale, find a book of tales (the Brothers Grimm are a good choice) and pick a story that appeals. Reread your story. Which image is the most powerful in the book? Again, choose art materials and paper. Depict your chosen image any way you like. You may even be drawn to use other materials, maybe making a model out of clay or scrap or natural objects such as sticks, stone or grasses. Once you've finished, look at your image. Think about how you feel when you see it. What does it remind you of? Write down your feelings or stray thoughts.

- **PAINT A DREAM** Dreams are also powerful ways to access our feelings. This is looked at in more depth in the Dreamworking section (Chapter 4), but it can be a good exercise to attempt painting an image from a dream, or trying to express the mood of a dream with paint or other art materials.

- **PAINT YOURSELF** How do you see yourself? Lay a huge sheet of paper on the floor. Lie down on it and ask someone to draw around your outline. Fill in the silhouette any way you want. You may want to cut out pictures from magazines or newspapers; you may prefer just to use colours. Are there any parts that feel 'cut off' (perhaps you feel drawn to get out the scissors and snip them away)? Are there any parts you don't want to colour in? Are there any parts that seem brighter, more 'real'? How does this exercise make you feel about your body?

12 Energy Therapies

Colour therapy

Researchers into the amazing world of colour have found that the colours we encounter – in our homes and our workplaces, in the clothes we wear and even in the foods we eat – can have enormous effects on our lives. Colour can affect health and happiness, success and our sex lives. Red walls in a pub or bar could mean more fights at closing time, while pink walls in a prison appear to make inmates quieter and less aggressive. People who wear a lot of blue may be on a constant diet yet never lose weight, while royal blue in a custody cell might urge criminals to come clean.

There is no doubt that colour sends out messages. 'It has been noted that 60 per cent of an individual's reaction to any situation is based on colour (surroundings, clothes etc.),' says colour therapist Marie Louise Lacy, 'so it is important to have the right colours in our environment, whether at home or at work.'

Psychologists have used colour as a form of personality testing for years; the colours we choose can give a very clear indication of our current state of mind. In 'chroma-totherapy', colour therapists use lamps with different coloured filters which flood the body with colour; some prescribe 'colour diets' or advise clients to dress in certain colours or decorate their houses in particular hues to heal an array of physical and emotional conditions. Practitioners of 'colourpuncture' beam coloured light onto precise points on the body.

A growing mass of solid scientific research seems to back the claims. Carlton Wagner, director of the Wagner Institute for Color Research in California, has shown that viewing certain colours triggers physical changes. Dr David Rainey, of John Carroll University in Ohio, agrees. He has found that seeing red can stimulate the glandular system and increase heart rate, blood pressure and respiration.

What can colour therapy help?

- Colour therapy is useful for centring people It is helpful in difficult situations such as bereavement, shock and dependency.
- It eases stress-related conditions and can soothe anxiety, depression and insomnia.
- Research into colourpuncture has shown it to be effective in treating children's insomnia, bronchitis and migraine.
- Practitioners of colourpuncture say it can help virtually any complaint and even help people overcome psychological trauma.

What can I expect from a session?

WHERE WILL I HAVE THE TREATMENT?
You will usually be lying on a couch In the therapist's room.

WILL I BE CLOTHED?
Yes, you will be fully clothed.

WHAT HAPPENS?
A colourpuncture session can last from 10 minutes to an hour depending on the problem. Before treatment, the practitioner will take a full case history and also a Kirlian photograph to gain an impression of the person's energy. On the basis of this, he or she will decide which points or areas to target and which colours to use out of the 200 or so in the colourpuncture repertory. You will then lie on a couch, and points (often on the face, back and feet) will be targeted with the colour puncture tool for between 30 and 60 seconds at a time. It's pleasant and deeply relaxing.

Chromatotherapists will beam a precise intensity of colour at the patient using large lamps or small torches, some employ a computer controlled instrument called a colour-form-rhythm beamer which transmits finely tuned intensities of colour, some may use coloured oils. Clients usually pick the oil that most appeals to them – a basic tenet of colour healing is that we intrinsically know what we need. The oil is then generally spritzed around the aura or at specific chakras. You may also be asked to visualize partic-ular colours (see below)

WILL IT HURT?
No, it doesn't hurt at all.

WILL ANYTHING STRANGE HAPPEN?
It is usually just very relaxing.

WILL I BE GIVEN ANYTHING TO TAKE?
No, but you may be asked to spritz yourself with coloured oils.

IS THERE ANY HOMEWORK?
You may be advised to wear certain colours or alter your surroudings to include different colours.

Do-it-yourself colour breathing

Lie down or sit in a comfortable chair and allow yourself to relax. Breathe comfortably and deeply, but keep the rhythm of your breathing natural and relaxed.

Now imagine yourself bathed in the colour you choose. As you breathe in, imagine the colour entering your body through your solar plexus (just above your abdomen) and spreading throughout your body. As you breathe out, visualize the complementary colour suffusing and leaving your body.

Blue relaxes and brings peace. Visualize blue when you can't go to sleep – it's great for insomnia. Use blue also when you can't stop to think calmly. Its complement is **orange**.

Green is the great healer. Use it to cleanse, to balance and to purify your system. It is useful if you continually take your work home with you or take your home worries to work. Green helps to keep thoughts in balance. Its complement is **magenta**.

Magenta is the great releaser. Breathe magenta when you need to let go of the past, of old thoughts and obsessions. It's wonderful as an aid during change, of whatever kind. It also brings out your spiritual energies. Its complement is **green**.

Orange is for fun, happiness and sheer joy. If you are feeling dull and gloomy, or fed up with your work, choose orange. Its complement is **blue**.

Red gives energy and vitality; it increases your strength and your sexuality. Use red when you lack energy, when you're so exhausted you can barely think. Its complement is **turquoise**.

Turquoise calms and soothes; it strengthens the immune system and can help feverish conditions and inflammations. Use turquoise if you feel dominated by other people or always give in to their thoughts and ideas. Its complement is **red**.

Violet is the colour of dignity and self-respect. Breathe it in when you feel lacking in self-esteem. Use it also when you find you are putting yourself down or start to feel that, no matter how hard you try, you will never do as well as others. Its complement is **yellow**.

Yellow is a wonderful colour for studying and concentrating, as it stimulates your intellectual and mental powers and increases your ability to be objective. It increases detachment and helps if you are feeling oversensitive or controlled by other people, or when you can't let go. Its complement is **violet**.

Flower and gem therapies

Flower and gem remedies are among the most remarkable healers known. They treat not physical symptoms as such, but the emotional states that underlie much illness and disharmony. They are gentle enough to use on tiny babies, yet powerful enough to produce profound shifts. Dr Edward Bach, a pioneer in the field, even brought people out of unconsciousness by using the remedies.

Numerous ancient cultures employed flowers to treat emotional states; some people even go so far as to claim that flower and gem essences were the ultimate healing systems in the highly evolved mythical cultures of Atlantis and Lemuria. Around 70 years ago, the British physician Dr Edward Bach established 38 remedies based on common trees and plants such as oak, walnut, clematis and mustard. Bach believed that the healing power of plants lies in their energy, an energy that can restore ailing bodies and souls. In order to tap that energy, he discovered, it was not necessary to ingest the whole plant (as in herbalism), but merely to take in the essence of the plant, captured by putting the flowers in a glass bowl of pure spring water and letting them steep in the sunlight for a few hours.

Practitioners believe that the remedies work by vibration. Apparently, the essences of flowers and gems vibrate at a very high level and so affect our bodies at the most subtle level. Rather than dealing with the dense matter of flesh and blood, the remedies go straight to the core of our being, working from the epicentre out to the denser fabric of the emotional and physical body.

In the past decade or so, other people have expanded the Bach system and now there are a host of various flower, tree and gem remedies. People the world over have discovered their native flowers and plants' healing properties: there are around 30 ranges of flower and gem essences from places as far afield as Australia, Alaska and the Himalayas.

What can flower and gem therapies help?

- Flower and gem essences will help any problem that has an emotional element.
- They have been used in conjunction with nutritional therapy to help people lose weight.
- They work wonderfully with children – helping to combat nightmares, fears, anxiety and exam nerves.
- Chronic depression responds well to these therapies, as do most psychological disorders.
- They can help with problems such as fears and phobias, uncertainty, doubt and anxiety
- Some remedies help with life shifts such as moving, marriage, having children, menopause, retirement and death of a loved one,

What can I expect from a session?

WHERE WILL I HAVE THE TREATMENT?
You will be sitting in a chair in the therapist's room.

WILL I BE CLOTHED?
Yes, you will be fully clothed.

WHAT HAPPENS?
Expect to be asked a lot of questions. It can be a lengthy process to find precisely the right remedies; a skilled practitioner will be looking for the underlying emotional blockages. Don't be surprised if the practitioner asks about any fears and concerns; about how you view yourself, the world and the people around you; or if you have any negative emotions; and so on.

Some practitioners combine these essences with other therapies, such as hypnotherapy, cranio-sacral therapy or more general psychotherapy. At the end of your session, the therapist will make up a bottle of remedies for you to take away with you.

WILL IT HURT?
No, it won't hurt physically. However, some people find the close questioning may bring up painful realizations.

WILL ANYTHING STRANGE HAPPEN?
It's unlikely that anything strange will happen during the session, but you may find quite sudden shifts occurring once you start taking the remedy.

WILL I BE GIVEN ANYTHING TO TAKE?
Yes, you will be given a bottle containing your remedies diluted in water and with a little brandy as preservative. You will take them (usually in water or other drinks) several times a day.

IS THERE ANY HOMEWORK?
No, you don't usually have anything else to do.

The Bach remedies at a glance

The Bach flower remedies are totally safe to self-administer. Simply add one or two drops of the remedy you feel you need to a glass of water and sip it throughout the day. Alternatively, you can make up a stock bottle containing several essences. Fill a 30 ml (1 fl oz) bottle three-quarters full with natural spring water. Add 2 drops each of your chosen remedies (you can use up to 5). Top up the bottle with a little brandy or cider vinegar for preservation. Shake well. Take at least 4 drops four times daily until the bottle is finished. These are the main personality traits associated with the 38 Bach flower remedies.

For fear – aspen (vague, undefined fears); mimulus (fear of known things – heights, spiders, etc.; cherry plum (irrational thoughts and fears); red chestnut (overanxiety and fear for others); rock rose (sheer terror, sudden shocks and alarm).

For uncertainty – cerato (doubting your judgment); gorse (hopelessness, pessimism); gentian (despondency, discouragement); hornbeam (lack of energy, listlessness); scleranthus (indecisiveness); wild oat (lack of direction in life, uncertainty about career).

For loneliness – impatiens (impatience); heather (self-obsession); water violet (aloofness, disdain).

For oversensitivity – agrimony (tortured thoughts hidden behind a cheerful façade); centaury (timidness, subservience); holly (envy, jealousy, hatred); walnut (difficulty adapting to change).

For despondency or despair – crab apple (self-disgust); elm (overwhelmed by responsibility); larch (lack of confidence); oak (struggling on against the odds); pine (guilt, self-blame); sweet chestnut (extreme despair); star of Bethlehem (after-effects of severe shock); willow (resentment).

For overconcern for others – beech (intolerance, need always to be right); chicory (selfishness, possessiveness); vervain (overenthusiastic, fanatical); vine (domineering); rock water (self-repression).

For insufficient interest in the present – chestnut bud (keep repeating same mistakes); clematis (daydreaming); honeysuckle (nostalgia); mustard (depression); olive (exhaustion, 'burn-out'); white chestnut (persistent worries); wild rose (resignation, apathy).

Light therapy

One dose of spring sunshine and the whole world seems to smile. Since time immemorial, people have valued the healing energy of light. From the earliest writings, we know that, among others, the Egyptians, the Greeks, the Romans and the Arabs all recognized the healing powers of sunlight. The modern history of light therapy as such starts in the nineteenth century, when natural sunlight was used as a cure for all kinds of ailments, from paralysis to tuberculosis. Modern research shows demonstrably that the pure sunlight of spring can have measurable, highly beneficial, effects on our health, both physiological and psychological.

Unfortunately, few of us take enough of this essential 'medicine'. Light therapists say that changes in our working lives mean that most of us are now seriously light deprived. In the past, we used to work on the land: now we work mainly indoors. An office may be warmer, drier and more comfortable than the average field, but it is also darker. Our offices are lit at between 200 and 1,000 lux (the measurement for light) when, in reality, we need levels around ten times brighter. The most common result is the well-documented syndrome of seasonal affective disorder (SAD), but light therapists reckon this is the tip of the iceberg: around 60 per cent of the population suffer in a less dramatic way. Lack of light can lead to depression and lethargy, disturbed sleep patterns and plummeting energy levels. Our metabolism can suffer; so, too, can our hormone levels. Even conditions such as osteoporosis and asthma worsen without regular doses of sunlight.

If we can't go out into the light, we have to bring the light in to us. SAD sufferers have used light boxes for some years now to help their symptoms, but recently a new brand of light therapy has been developed which promises benefits for virtually everyone. This new light reproduces as closely as possible the pure spring light of the northern hemisphere, the clear, soft gleam that so revitalizes us, body and soul. In practical terms, it's a combination of fluorescent tubes that gives out the whole spectrum of wavelengths in natural daylight, except the harmful ultraviolet (UVB) rays that can cause burning and skin cancer.

What can light therapy help?

- Light therapy increases energy levels.
- It can help with many types of depression.
- A mere 20 minutes of light therapy can apparently lower blood pressure for up to a week and will also lower blood cholesterol levels.
- Light therapy balances hormones, so it can be used as an alternative to hormone replacement therapy (HRT) and also to increase fertility.
- Full-spectrum light can kill bacteria and accelerate wound healing.
- Exposure to the lights increases the production of vitamin D in the body, which in turn improves the absorption of calcium, phosphorus and magnesium, making light therapy useful in cases of arthritis, osteoporosis and dental caries.
- As daylight suppresses the production of melatonin (which helps send us to sleep), light therapy can be used to treat sleep disorders and jet lag with great success.

What can I expect from a session?

WHERE WILL I HAVE THE TREATMENT?
You will be lying on a comfortable couch.

WILL I BE CLOTHED?
You can wear as much or little clothing as you like.

WHAT HAPPENS?
First, a detailed medical history will be taken. You will then be asked to take off your shoes and as much clothing as you wish, and to lie on the couch. Any glasses or contact lenses

must be removed because the light can only reach the pineal gland (essential for hormonal balance) through the eyes.

The lights are mounted in a panel above the couch several feet above your body – they look much like a sunbed, except that the centre tubes are a beautiful shade of blue. For the best effects, you keep your eyes open (although you don't have to look directly at the light) for the first 20 minutes.

WILL IT HURT
No, it's absolutely painless – in fact, you won't feel anything at all except pleasantly warm and relaxed.

WILL ANYTHING STRANGE HAPPEN?
No, nothing strange occurs with this therapy.

WILL I BE GIVEN ANYTHING TO TAKE?
No, medication is not a part of the treatment.

IS THERE ANY HOMEWORK?
No, there's no need to do anything at home.

Bright ideas to bring sunlight into your life

Lightbathing, say light therapists, stimulates the circulation, tones up muscles, detoxifies the body and boosts production of vitamin D and hormones. Here are some tips on simple ways to maximize your light exposure.

• At times of the year when the danger of burning is very low, get as much natural daylight as you can. There is no need to lie exposed to the sun – gardening, dog-walking or even just walking outside in your lunch hour can help.
• As the sun gets brighter, you need to adjust the amount of sun you take to suit your skin type. Light therapists insist that it is burning that causes skin cancer, not sensible exposure. As a rough guide, you need to stay out for half the amount of time that you can safely be in the sun before burning, that will be around 10 minutes in very bright sunlight for very fair skins, through to an hour for people with very dark-toned skins.
• The more of your skin that is exposed to the light the better.
• Glasses, sunglasses and contact lenses all filter out the light. Wearing dark glasses all the time, say light therapists, will tend to make you depressed or irritable – use a hat instead to shield you from glare.

Metamorphic technique

The metamorphic technique is neither a therapy nor a massage. It's not healing and nor, its practitioners insist, is it even a treatment. Of all the practices in complementary medicine, this is perhaps the most mystical and unexplained. Yet, nebulous though it may appear, thousands of people who have experienced the technique affirm that life is never the same once you step onto the metamorphic path.

The metamorphic technique was developed in the 1960s while naturopath and reflex-ologist Robert St John was working in a school for mentally challenged children. Although his work did seem to be helping the children, the changes were, to his mind, not deep or lasting enough. He wanted something that would change the children for the better permanently. While practising reflexology, he came to the conclusion that not only are all the parts of the body represented in the foot (as reflexology teaches), but also that our passage through the womb, from conception to birth, is mapped out on the side of the foot, along the points reflexologists call the spinal reflexes. His finding, in itself, would be merely a curiosity were it not for the fact that St John also came to believe that the ailments we suffer and the characteristics we carry through life are established during the gestation period, in our mothers' wombs. By working on the feet with a particular light touch, he found he could release blocks and facilitate 'transformations' on both a physical and an emotional level.

In 1979, the Metamorphic Association was set up as a registered charity to promote the theory worldwide. Despite testimonials from both orthodox doctors and complementary practitioners, clinics, schools and institutions, practitioners claim it is not the technique itself nor the practitioner which brings about such results: it is the life force working inside the person. It's hard to see how such a simple technique can instigate profound changes, but people swear it has transformed their lives. Some find new relationships or end outdated ones; some move house or change their jobs; others are prompted to pursue a healthier lifestyle or to seek medical advice.

Although the philosophy of metamorphosis is esoteric, the practice is remarkably simple. It can be done by anyone and there is no need to go into deep meditation – you can talk or watch television while you are doing it.

What can metamorphic technique help?

- People attest that metamorphosis has helped them change their lives – it provides the impetus to make profound shifts.
- If given during pregnancy and labour, it can ease labour; many midwives are now learning the technique.
- Babies and young children react very well – it calms and soothes them.
- It can help families bond and to become more of a unit.
- It has been given to people with HIV and AIDS, and taught to their friends and family.
- Metamorphic technique is used a lot with children who are physically or mentally challenged, or have learning difficulties.
- Some people have introduced the metamorphic technique into use in hospitals, hospices and jails.

What can I expect from a session?

WHERE WILL I HAVE THE TREATMENT?
You will be sitting in or lying on a comfortable chair or couch.

WILL I BE CLOTHED?
Yes, you just take off your shoes and socks.

WHAT HAPPENS?
You won't be asked for any details about your life. You are simply invited to remove your shoes and socks, and sit in or lie on a relaxing chair or couch. The practitioner then takes your foot and starts to work. The touch is light and fluid; sometimes it feels as if your foot is being gently polished; at others, it is as if the practitioner were searching for something. Occasionally, he or she may yawn, sneeze or even burp — this is caused by blockages

passing through the practitioner's hands into his or her body. Yawning, sneezing or even burping apparently allows the blocks to disappear harmlessly into the air.

After working on both feet, the practitioner works on your hands and then finally on your head, leaving you feeling very relaxed yet surprisingly energized.

WILL IT HURT?
No, It's totally painless and very pleasant.

WILL ANYTHING STRANGE HAPPEN?
Not usually, but some people report that, during a session, they 'see' scenes from their lives or that they re-experience emotions that they felt when they were in the womb.

WILL I BE GIVEN ANYTHING TO TAKE?
No, medication is not part of the treatment.

IS THERE ANY HOMEWORK?
There is any specific homework, although many people learn the technique for use on family and friends. Even though the philosophy of metamorphic technique is a rather esoteric one, the actual practice is remarkably simple. It can be learned over a weekend (the basic touch can be taught in just 5 minutes). Absolutely anyone can learn to practise the metamorphic technique and you can even talk or watch television while doing it. The Metamorphic Association is particularly keen to teach parents this technique, as it believes it can help to bond families together and allow them to move and transform as a unit, a functioning whole, rather than as individuals.

Reiki

Reiki, the Japanese art of spiritual healing, is mysterious and inscrutable. Contradictions abound as to its purpose and practice. Some practitioners call reiki 'relaxation therapy'; others insist it can be far from relaxing. Although it is known as 'healing', its exponents freely admit that sometimes reiki chooses not to heal. Reiki, in its truest form, is far more than just a system of healing – it is a profound spiritual path. The word *reiki* is made up of two words: *ki* is the life force (the Japanese equivalent of the Chinese qi or chi that flows through the meridians), while the word *rei* means spiritually guided.

Reiki was 'discovered' by a Japanese man called Mikao Usui around the beginning of the twentieth century. After a 14-year search for the secret of physical healing, Usui found the 'answer' in an ancient sutra or sacred text in a Zen monastery. In the manner of all the best yarns, no one since then has been able to rediscover the precise text, but it led him to meditate on a mountain where he was shown a vision of four symbols which could be used for healing. Coming down the mountain, Usui stumbled and hurt his toe. When he placed his hand on the foot, the injury healed – and he realized his quest was over.

The physical part of the reiki system is very simple. Consisting of 20 'holds', it can be learnt in a weekend. There is no need to learn anatomy or physiology; students aren't expected to study even basic psychology. The key is in the spiritual symbols which are 'transmitted' to the trainee healer. Then, it seems, the healing force is free to flow through. Practitioners insist it is not they who are healing; it is not even the reiki which heals. Rather, it is the individual who is being treated who decides how much of the healing energy to take and use.

Currently, reiki is big business. There are countless workshops promising to transform you into a reiki 'master' in a weekend or two. Frankly, they smack a little of pyramid selling and I would urge you to find someone who has followed the reiki way of life for many years and slowly gained their attunement.

What can reiki help?

- Practitioners do not promise to heal anything through reiki – rather, the body will choose what to do with the energy and may heal itself or may not.
- Many people have it simply for deep relaxation and stress relief.
- It is often used as a tool for self-development and spiritual questing.
- Studies have shown that reiki can hasten healing after injuries.
- There have been cases of 'miraculous' cures – tumours disappearing, wounds healing, illnesses vanishing, long-term depression lifting. Practitioners are adamant, however, that they can make no claims.
- Reiki is practised extensively in hospices, especially with cancer patients. Sometimes people go into remission; sometimes they die, but in peace — without fear and feeling calm and accepting.

What can I expect from a session?

WHERE WILL I HAVE THE TREATMENT?
You will be lying on a couch.

WILL I BE CLOTHED?
Yes, you will remain fully clothed throughout.

WHAT HAPPENS?
It's up to you whether you talk to the practitioner or not – you can tell them any problems or simply keep your counsel. However, you will be asked if you are on any medication, particularly insulin. The reason is that diabetics need to be carefully monitored after reiki because sometimes the amounts of insulin they need decline sharply. The same can be true for dosages of other medication.

You lie fully clothed on a massage table, with soft Oriental music playing in the background. The practitioner begins by gently but firmly touching your head with his or her fingers. After several minutes, he or she will lift one hand and touch another part of your head, then the other hand follows. So it continues as the practitioner works down your body.

You will find yourself becoming more and more relaxed, and probably quite drowsy. It's not uncommon to fall fast asleep while lying on the couch. Time becomes quite fluid and it can be hard to tell whether 5 minutes or 50 have passed. After an hour (the usual length of most sessions), you will be gently 'brought to' by the practitioner, who will usually leave you alone for a while to bring yourself hack to full waking awareness.

Don't be surprised if you find you feel emotional after a session: it's not uncommon to feel sadness, anger or intense joy. Many practitioners will sit and talk with you about your experiences (often over a cup of herbal tea).

WILL IT HURT?
No, it is completely painless.

WILL ANYTHING STRANGE HAPPEN?

You may well 'see' past scenes from your life. Your limbs may spontaneously convulse or twitch. You may also find that, after a while, you can't feel the practitioner's hands on you or you don't know exactly where they are. Some people see brilliant colours or feel a burning sensation from the hands during a reiki session. Others feel nothing at all.

WILL I BE GIVEN ANYTHING TO TAKE?

No, medication is not part of the treatment.

IS THERE ANY HOMEWORK?

No, although a lot of people do go on to learn reiki so that they can practise it on their family and friends.

Do-it-yourself reiki

The heart of reiki is spiritual. Although the actual holds are easily learned, you need to have the spiritual symbols 'transmitted' to you before true reiki healing energy can flow. However, this breathing and touching exercise gives a taste of the reiki touch. You will feel more calm, centred and relaxed. Find a time when you won't be disturbed to practise this exercise for best results.

1 Lie on your back, make yourself comfortable and close your eyes. Start paying attention to your breath and follow its rhythm, noticing how it flows in and out.

2 Now put your hands on your body wherever you feel drawn to or where you feel tension. Drawn on your intuition to locate the spot in your body that needs relaxation the most.

3 Now direct your breath to this place. Imagine you are breathing into that place. Visualize your breath as universal life energy that is flowing through you. Imagine it collecting and expanding under your hands. Notice the feeling of relaxation and peace as it gradually spreads from that place beneath your hands throughout your entire body.

4 After about 5 minutes, place your hands on another part of your body and repeat step 3. You may find that your breathing changes with this place. If so, just notice it and continue.

5 Now move on to two further places in your body and charge them with revitalizing energy.

6 Slowly open your eyes, stretch and return to normal consciousness.

Sound therapy

A soprano can break a glass by matching its vibration. You can bring down a bridge by stamping over it in rhythm. So, the reasoning goes that, if you can destroy with sound, then there is no reason why you can't heal with sound.

Simply making different sounds can affect your mood in minutes. Listening to powerful chants can affect both body and mind. Sound researchers believe that sound could be the medicine of the future.

'Disease is simply part of our body vibrating out of tune,' says pioneering sound therapist Jonathan Goldman. He explains that, 'Every organ, bone, tissue and other part of the body has a healthy resonant frequency. When that frequency alters, that part of the body vibrates out of harmony and that is what is termed disease. If it were possible to determine the correct frequency for a healthy organ and then project it into that part which is diseased, the organ should return to its normal frequency and a healing should occur.'

By creating sounds which are harmonious with the 'correct' frequency of our organs, we could all learn how to heal ourselves. Goldman and other sound researchers have been focusing most of their attention on the sacred chants of varying traditions, believing that the incredible harmonics which most of them share could have profound effects on body and mind.

Dr Alfred Tomatis, a French physician and researcher, found that Gregorian chants can have a neurophysical effect which charges the brain and stimulates the central nervous system. American researchers found that harmonic sounds reduced respiration and heart rate, relaxing the entire body and mind. Apparently when sound healing is taking place, a process called 'entrainment' occurs: everything within the body that has a rhythm (heartbeat, respiration, brainwaves, movement in the intestine, etc.) starts to change in order to synchronize with the rhythm of a more powerful body – the healer.

What can sound therapy help?

- Sound therapy can increase confidence.
- It can alleviate stress and help stress-related illnesses.
- It Increases energy and wellbeing, and can be deeply relaxing.
- It can help dissipate headaches and prevent migraine.
- Many people use it as a tool for personal or spiritual growth.

What can I expect from a session?

WHERE WILL I HAVE THE TREATMENT?
You will be treated in the sound therapist's room.

WILL I BE CLOTHED?
Yes, you will be fully clothed.

WHAT HAPPENS?
An experienced sound therapist directs sounds at your body either working through the major chakras or focusing on specific organs or parts of the body. You simply stand still with your eyes shut while he or she projects the sound at you. This can feel incredible, like being doused with a cool shower of sound. You may also be taught how to make healing sounds, or toning, yourself.

The aim is not to make perfect sounds – in fact, it doesn't even matter if you are tone deaf. Many people go on to learn sound healing at workshops, where participants are taken through simple exercises as part of a group.

WILL IT HURT?
No, it doesn't hurt at all.

WILL ANYTHING STRANGE HAPPEN?
When sound is directed at you, it's not uncommon to feel surges of energy through your body. Some people say they feel a hum in their bones and explosions in their heads.

WILL I BE GIVEN ANYTHING TO TAKE?
No, medication is not part of the treatment.

IS THERE ANY HOMEWORK?
Yes, ideally you should practise making sounds and toning at home.

Do-it-yourself sound techniques

- Humming is a great way to calm yourself. If you're feeling anxious, stressed or nervous, just sit quietly and hum very gently. Feel the hum resonating through your body. Where can you feel it? Does it change if you alter the note of the hum?
- Exaggerated yawning is ideal if you're feeling tired. We hold a lot of tension in our jaws and mouths, so stretching the mouth therefore reduces tension. Give your body a good stretch as well to wake it up.
- If you're feeling irritable and tense, try an elongated, noisy sigh. Groaning, too, can help release negative emotions. Forget about being polite – really let go.
- Take every opportunity to sing. Sing along with the radio, while you're doing house-work, in the bath (of course!) and while you're driving in the car. Don't worry about what your voice sounds like – just belt it out.
- Try toning the different vowel sounds – ah, eh, iii, oh, uh. Where can you feel them in your body? How do these sounds make you feel?
- Play with mantras. They don't have to be 'ohm' or anything spiritual – simply try singing positive statements, repeating them with different tunes. If you're feeling tense, try singing: 'I'm calm, I'm calm, I'm really, really calm.'
- Experiment with listening to different kinds of music and work out what effect each one has on your mood. Try listening to some of the sacred chants – Gregorian, Tibetan, Mongolian overtone chanting, etc.

Part 2 *Soul*

What is a soul? We can touch our bodies, but no one has ever actually touched a soul. We can sense our minds working, we can feel our emotions, but our soul is somehow far more ineffable. Many mystical traditions hold that the soul is the part of us that is divine and eternal. When our bodies have turned to dust and our minds are no more, we exist as pure soul. But exactly what does that mean in daily life?

I think you can sense your soul and, with practice, you can become more and more aware of it and its needs. Think of a time when you were overcome with wonder, with love or beauty. It could be the sight of a newborn baby gazing up at you. It might be the vision of a sunrise or sunset, when the earth is bathed in breathtaking beauty. It could be the majesty of a mountain range or the tiny miracle of a snowdrop pushing through the rock-solid frozen earth. It might just be a warm feeling as you sit listening to your friends chatting or a sense of peace as you quietly muse on your own. At these, and other, moments, we catch a glimpse of our souls – we feel an inkling of something deep within that is not caught up in the day-to-day detritus of life.

The aim of this section is to find simple, effective ways by which we can nurture this relationship with our souls. If we want to get the most out of our lives, to feel fulfilled, exhilarated and peaceful, we need to address our soul just as much as our bodily and psychological requirements. In some ways, the soul connection is the most important. If your soul is in good form, everything else should fall into place because we find soul everywhere – in the incredible entity we call a body, in the halls of our minds, in nature, in our work, in our personal lives, in our sexuality, in our dreams. We explore our souls both in the joyful moments and in the dark abysses of depression, fear, sorrow and anger.

As we come to recognize our souls, we may even feel the tug towards something larger, more wise and powerful than us: we start to feel our connection to Spirit. In the past, the most common way to explore this was through organized religion. This is still a valid path and one we look at in the first part of this section. However, we don't just find our connection to Spirit and 'God' within a church or mosque, a synagogue or temple, so we will also be looking at alternative ways to find a sense of unity with Spirit.

13 The Spiritual Traditions

There are many paths to the Divine. Some people grow up with one particular religion and it resonates so deeply within their souls that they follow it all their lives. In many ways, they are the lucky ones. They have a certainty about their spiritual lives that can be deeply comforting and reassuring. For other people, finding the right path can be a long and often painful process. Sometimes it entails long periods of searching and experimenting – often accompanied by intense disappointment. If this applies to you, don't be discouraged. The journey may be difficult, but we all tend to get there in the end.

The 'standard' religions have a weight, tradition and power that can make them deeply welcoming. They are not, however, the only way. Today, many people are rediscovering ancient religious traditions such as shamanism or Wicca and paganism. Still others will feel drawn to forge an individual relationship with Spirit. Go with your heart, listen to your soul. Truly, it doesn't matter whether you find God (Goddess, Supreme Creator, whatever it is that underpins the universe) in a babbling brook or in the vaults of a cathedral. All that is important is that your spirituality soothes your soul, that it has meaning for you and that it brings you peace.

In this section, we will look briefly at some of the great spiritual traditions of the world.

Christianity

Christianity is the world's largest religion – about a third of the world's population regard themselves as Christians, although Islam is projected to become the dominant religion during this century.

In general, all Christians follow the teachings of Jesus Christ, a Jewish preacher born c 7–4 BCE. Most Christians regard Jesus as the son of God and one of the Holy Trinity (Father, Son and Holy Spirit) who was incarnated as a man, born of a virgin (Mary). He preached God's word before being condemned to death and crucified. On the third day after his death, Jesus was resurrected and ascended to heaven.

There is a wide divergence between the teachings and beliefs of the various Christian sects. Some believe that we are born fundamentally sinful and that we can only be 'saved' from hell and damnation through a life of repentance and prayer. Others are far less judgmental and consider the concept of hell as symbolic, rather than an actual location for eternal torment and punishment. At its most simple, Christianity really comes down to two tenets: love God and be kind to others.

Prayer is the most common form of worship. In the past, retreats and pilgrimage, alongside fasting and meditative techniques, were part of Christianity and many people are now returning to these practices. There is also renewed interest in the varying forms of Christian mysticism, such as Gnosticism, and in the wisdom of early Christian mystics and sages such as Hildegaard of Bingen and Meister Eckhart.

Christian mysticism emphasizes the relationship between man and God, and also God and the world – teaching that God can be found within us and also in the world around us. Through diligent practice, we can obtain a sense of oneness with God. As Hildegaard of Bingen put it: 'The mystery of God hugs you in its all-encompassing arms.'

Islam

Note: Muslims always follow the name of the prophet Muhammad with the words 'peace be upon him'; when written, this is abbreviated to 'pbuh'. As a mark of respect, we have followed this practice.

Islam is the second-largest world religion – and it is expanding very fast. It is also the youngest of the world's great religions. Islam is generally believed to have been founded in 622 CE by the prophet Muhammad (pbuh). Muhammad (pbuh) was raised in the desert but travelled widely, meeting people of a wide variety of religious beliefs. At the age of 40, in 610 BCE, he received divine revelations from the angel Jibreel (or Gabriel) while he was in Mecca. He was given the task of converting his people from their pagan, polytheistic beliefs and what he saw as their moral decadence and materialism.

Muhammad (pbuh) taught that we need to relinquish our selfish individual needs and personal will, surrendering instead to the divine will of God – the word *Islam* means 'surrender'. These revelations, the divine words of God, were written down and became the Qur'an, the divine scripture, or writings, that all Muslims follow. The Hadith, a collection of the sayings of the prophet Muhammad (pbuh), is used as an additional guide for living.

The principle of 'surrender' is readily demonstrated by a Sufi (see below) teaching story in which a man knocks on God's door. 'Who's there?' comes the voice of God from inside. 'It's me,' says the man. 'Well, go away,' says God, 'there's no room in here for two.' The man walked away and wandered around alone in the desert until he realized his mistake. He then returned to the door and knocked again. Once again, God asked, 'Who's there?' This time the man answered, 'You.' 'Then come in,' replied God.

Muslims have a series of duties including regular prayer, charitable donations, fasting and pilgrimage. Perhaps most often misunderstood is the concept of Jihad (struggle). While some fundamentalist Muslims have seen it as a literal call to enforce conversion to their faith, via crusades and bloodshed, the vast majority of Muslims see it as a personal, internal battle, a struggle with one's self.

Islam is a very moral religion: devout Muslims reject alcohol, gambling and the taking of drugs. They recognize Jesus, but regard him as a prophet, rather than a deity. Other prophets such as Abraham and Moses are also respected. Muhammad (pbuh) is seen as the last of the prophets.

There are several strands of Islam. One which is gaining popularity in the West is Sufism. This is a highly mystical path, characterized by its profoundly beautiful spiritual poetry which talks about the longing for union with God and often expresses this in 'romantic' terms, with God as the deeply Beloved with whom the Sufi shares an intoxicating and passionate sacred love.

Hinduism

Despite its great antiquity, Hinduism remains a vibrant faith today and is the world's third-largest religion. It is said to have originated in the Indus Valley around 4000 to 2200 BCE.

There are literally thousands of different strands of Hinduism and, to the novice, it may seem very confusing and even contradictory, with different sects worshipping a variety of deities. There is, however, basically one eternal truth: we are all part of God and God is within each of us. 'Atman is Brahman' means the Higher Self (our true spiritual identity, rather than our common ego) is God: our consciousness is simply an expression of the cosmic consciousness.

The Hindu sage Ramakrishna said: 'The ego is like a stick dividing water into two. It creates the impression that you are one and I am another. When the ego vanishes, you will realize that Brahman is your own inner Consciousness.'

Although the entire universe is experienced as one divine entity, this deity is also expressed as a trinity: Brahma (the Creator, who continues to create new realities), Vishnu or Krishna (the Preserver, who preserves these creations) and Shiva (the Destroyer, who can destroy, but be compassionate as well). Humans are seen as being trapped in samsara, a meaningless cycle of birth, life, death and rebirth. Karma (the accumulated sum of our good and bad deeds in life) will determine how we live our next life. The aim is to live as pure a life as possible so we can be reborn at a higher level and eventually achieve enlightenment and escape samsara.

There are various paths towards spiritual enlightenment, known as *yogas*. The hatha yoga we do as exercise was originally a path towards God through mastery of body and mind. Tantric yoga was initially a difficult path towards union with God through precise use of sexual energy. Other forms of yoga include bhakti yoga (which emphasizes prayer, worship and devotion) and gnana yoga (which is more intellectual, focusing on meditation, study of scripture and philosophy). Many Hindu practices are now used widely in the West, such as meditation, physical yoga and pranayama (breathing).

Buddhism

Buddhism was founded in Northern India, inspired by an Indian sage called Siddhartha Guatama, or simply Buddha, who was born in 563 BCE. At the age of 29, he left his family and career in order to seek truth. In 535 BCE, Siddhartha reached enlightenment and assumed the title of Buddha (which means 'One who has been awakened').

Buddhism has become enormously popular in the West in recent years – probably because of the extreme simplicity and clarity of its teachings. There is no belief in a 'God' as such, no need for personal saviours.

Buddhism teaches that we suffer because we fear death. Yet, in truth, there is no death because there is no separate 'self' to die. We are not individual souls, but all part of an indivisible whole. Our problems stem from the illusion (samsara) of our separation. The principal aim of Buddhism is to experience nirvana, the blissful state of enlightenment in which we are one with all of creation, all of consciousness.

Of course, the ego can have trouble with this philosophy – particularly the notion that each of us is like a drop of water which will eventually be absorbed back into the infinite ocean. Buddhists, however, insist that enlightenment is actually incredibly comforting, bringing the certain knowledge that our essential beings will never die.

Many Buddhist practices are also finding general favour today. Mindfulness (see pages 14–16) is a classic Buddhist practice. Meditation is used, too, and some Buddhists practise chanting, pilgrimage, ceremony and rituals.

Zen Buddhism is a form of Buddhism mingled with some elements of Taoism (see page 86). Founded in the sixth century CE by an Indian Buddhist, Bodhidharma, its aim is for us to discover who we are: to experience our true 'Buddha nature' in the emptiness of mind. In this state of 'empty mind', we have no sense of ourselves as individuals, but rather as part of the greater consciousness. Classic Zen practice is 'sitting', meditation's most basic form. Zen is also famous for the bizarre and seemingly illogical advice and practices of its masters, who seek to shock the mind into spiritual realization. A classic example is: 'What is your original face?' Such questions defeat the rational mind and may ultimately cause the seeker to stop striving and purely 'see'.

Judaism

Note: it is forbidden for Jews to spell the name of the deity in full, so they write 'G-d'. As a mark of respect, this practice has been followed here.

Judaism was founded around 2000 BCE when the G-d of the ancient people of Israel established a divine covenant with Abraham, making him the patriarch of many nations. He was followed by the patriarchs Isaac and Jacob. Moses was the next great leader of the ancient Israelites; he led the people out of captivity in Egypt and received the Law from G-d. There are around 18 million Jews in the world, mainly in the USA (around 7 million) and Israel (4.5 million).

There are two main books of scriptures. The Tanakh consists of three groups of books: the Torah (which contains Genesis, Exodus, Leviticus, Numbers and Deuteronomy); the Nevi'im (the Prophetic books of Isaiah, Amos, etc.) and the Ketuvim (the Writings, including Kings, Chronicles, etc.). The Talmud contains stories, laws, moral debates and medical knowledge, and is composed of material from two sources: the Mishnah (six 'orders' containing series of laws from the Hebrew scriptures) and the Gemara (including comments from hundreds of rabbis from 200–500 CE). The Gemara explains the Mishnah with other historical, sociological, legal and religious material.

Judaism teaches that there is only one G-d, who is Creator of everything and is without body. The entire world is seen as inherently good and its people basically good, creations of G-d. Believers can come closer to G-d by following the divine commandments. There is no saviour needed nor any other intermediaries. G-d communicates to the Jewish people through prophets and monitors people's behaviour, rewarding them for good deeds and punishing evil. One's actions are seen as very important and Jewish life is regulated by a large body of law – basically, the Ten Commandments of Moses are a synopsis of the Law (in all, there are 613 commandments found in Leviticus and other books).

Judaism celebrates a wide variety of festivals and regular worship is also expected. Prayer and study are an intrinsic part of Jewish life. Recently, many Westerners have become fascinated by the esoteric branch of Judaism, the Quabalah.

Taoism

The word *Tao* (pronounced 'dow', to rhyme with 'now') roughly translates as 'path', or 'the way'. The Tao is considered to be the force, or energy, which moves through and within all things in the universe. A deep mystical concept, the Tao can signify pure consciousness, an emptiness which is yet full or supreme oneness with creation. It is also seen in more prosaic terms as the way things are, the way life works.

The founder of Taoism was Lao-Tse (604–531 BCE), who was a contemporary of Confucius. He sought a way of avoiding the persistent warfare that plagued society and wrote down his ideas in a book, the Tao Te Ching, which is a combination of psychology and philosophy.

Taoism became a religious faith in 440 CE, when it was adopted as a state religion in China and Lao-Tse became venerated as a deity. Sadly, much of the Taoist heritage was destroyed during China's Cultural Revolution, instituted by China's former Communist leader Mao Tse-tung in 1966. Today, there are around 20 million practising Taoists and interest in the Tao is growing as people discover its concepts, often through acupuncture, tai chi, feng shui and the I Ching.

The goal of the Taoist is to become one with the Tao, the essential life energy of the universe. Understanding and wisdom are achieved not by prayer to a deity, but through observation of the world and its signs, inner contemplation and meditation. The world is seen as divided into two opposites – yin and yang – which should be kept in perfect balance. We humans, however, usually manage to upset this balance and one or other will become dominant, causing disharmony, disease and disturbance. Taoists strive to care for their bodies as well as their souls. It is considered essential to nurture one's qi (vital energy) and to keep yin and yang in balance. Similarly, one should develop virtue: seeking compassion, moderation and humility. Kindness is seen as a great virtue, as is careful planning and forethought.

One of the key concepts of Taoism is wu wei, achieving action through minimal effort, popularized in the West by the psychologist Carl Jung. Wu wei is explained as follows: it is the practice of going against the stream not by struggling against it and thrashing about, but by standing still and letting the stream do all the work.

Jainism (jain dharma)

Jainism traces its roots to the 24 Jinas (literally meaning 'those who overcame') in ancient East India. The first Jina was supposedly a giant who lived around eight and a half million years ago. The most recent, and last, Jina was Vardhamana, or Mahavira, who was born in 550 BCE and founded the Jain community. It took 13 years of deprivation for him to achieve enlightenment and, in 420 BCE, he starved himself to death. Jainism contains many elements in common with Hinduism and Buddhism, although it is far more ascetic. The world's four million Jains live almost entirely in India. Jainism teaches that the universe is without beginning or end; it exists as a series of layers:

- the supreme abode where the Siddha or liberated souls live
- the upper world: heavens where celestial beings live
- the middle world: earth and the rest of the universe
- the nether world: seven hells with various levels of punishment
- the nigoda: where the lowest forms of life reside

- universe space: layers of cloud surrounding the upper world of celestial beings
- space beyond: an infinite zone without soul, matter, time, motion or rest

We are all bound by karma, and moksha (liberation from constant reincarnation) is only achieved by enlightenment (which, in turn, can only be achieved by the harshest forms of ascetic living). There are five essential principles for life:

- **AHIMSA** This is basically non-violence. It is taken to the most extreme form – you must not commit mental, verbal or physical violence on any living thing, even an insect or vegetable. Jains consume only what will not kill the plant or animal from which it is taken – i.e. milk, fruit and nuts.
- **SATYA** This is speaking the truth always.
- **ASTEYA** This means not stealing.
- **BRAHMA-CHARYA** This is the soul's conduct – remaining faithful to one's spouse.
- **APARIGRAHA** This means detachment from people, places and material things. Some Jains even go as far as to reject clothing and go naked at all times.

Confucianism

Confucianism is not a religion as such, but more a series of codes of moral conduct. It was founded by K'ung Fu Tzu (commonly known as Confucius in English). He was not a prophet or philosopher, but, as he liked to put it, a 'transmitter', relaying the wisdom of the ancients. K'ung Fu Tzu was born in 551 BCE, in what is now the Shantung province of China. His writings are mainly concerned with morality, ethics and the proper use of political power. During his life, Confucius wandered through China accompanied by a small band of students; he spent his last years teaching in his homeland.

There are around six million Confucians in the world today. Many combine the ethical teaching of Confucianism with Taoist and Buddhist beliefs. The major ethical beliefs of Confucius include:

- **LI** Ritual, correct ways of behaving
- **HSIAO** Family values – love between parents and children, siblings, grandparents etc.
- **YI** Righteousness
- **XIN** Honesty and trustworthiness
- **JEN** Benevolence, kindness to others
- **CHUNG** Loyalty to the state

The Confucian tradition recognizes four major life passages, which are governed by ritual and celebration:

- **BIRTH** The spirit of the foetus (the T'ai-shen) is believed to protect the expectant mother and deal harshly with anyone who bothers her. There is a Confucian ritual for disposing of the placenta after birth and the new mother is made to rest and carefully fed a special diet for a month following the birth.
- **ATTAINING MATURITY** A group family meal of chicken celebrates the transition to adulthood.
- **MARRIAGE** An elaborate six-stage celebration takes place which involves minutely observed rituals for proposal, engagement, dowry, procession, marriage and reception, and, finally, morning after (breakfast).
- **DEATH** A willow branch is carried to the cemetery in order to symbolize the soul of the person who has died. Mourners contribute to the cost of the funeral and liturgies are performed on set dates for the first three years after death.

Shinto

Shinto was founded in Japan in around 500 BCE (or possibly earlier). It was originally a form of shamanism featuring nature and ancestor worship, divination and fertility cults. The word *shinto* comes from the Chinese *Shin Tao* ('Way of the Gods'). It was, and remains, a loosely based religion, with no written scriptures as such (although there are valued texts), no real figureheads and no body of religious law. Many Japanese follow both Buddhism and Shinto – in Shinto, Buddha is seen as another Kami or nature deity, and Buddhists in Japan regard the Kami as manifestations of Buddhas.

There are a large number of Kami, emanating from the original 'divine couple', Izanagi-no-mikoto and Izanami-no-mikoto, who gave birth to the Japanese islands. Their offspring became the various clan deities. Amaterasu, the Sun Goddess, was one of their daughters and is regarded as a chief deity. Many others are related to natural objects and creatures. There are guardian Kami in particular areas and locations; clans also have their particular protective Kami. The Kami are generally seen as benign protectors.

All of humanity is regarded as 'Kami's child' and hence sacred. So, too, is nature – to be close to nature is thus seen as being close to the gods; natural objects are often worshipped as sacred spirits. Ancestor worship is an integral part of Shinto and family life is very important – the main celebrations and rituals are all to do with family, birth and marriage. A strong emphasis is put on morality, cleanliness and kindness.

There is much of interest in Shinto for modern spiritual seekers and many of its practices are being taken up, in particular by those who practise Wicca, shamanism and druidism. Seasonal celebrations are a strong part of Shinto and there is a tradition of venerating sacred places, such as springs, mountains and trees. Ritual dance is common. Shinto believers make shrines and altars both within the home and in nature. They also visit communal shrines for celebrations and rituals. Charms are made and worn for healing and protection. Origami (literally, 'paper of the spirits') is about much more than making pretty shapes out of paper: it is made as a gift to spirits and placed on or around Shinto shrines. The paper is folded, rather than cut, out of respect for the tree spirit that gave its life to make the paper.

Sikhism

Many people regard Sikhism as a Hindu cult, but, although it does contain elements of Hinduism (as well as Islam), Sikhism is fundamentally different and unique. *Sikh* means 'learner' and it was founded by Shri Guru Nanak Dev Ji (1469–1538), who was born in the Punjab. He received a vision in which he was instructed to preach the way to enlightenment and God.

There are around 22.5 million Sikhs worldwide. Their goal is to build a close, loving relationship with God. This is seen as almost akin to that of a bride longing for her husband. God is regarded as a powerful yet totally compassionate entity. He is present in everything, from the greatest spiritual seeker to the lowliest grub. There is one God who alone should be worshipped, but, as with Islam, He has many names. Sikhs do not deny the other gods of Hindu belief, but consider them lesser gods who should not be worshipped. Like Hindus and Buddhists, they believe in karma and reincarnation. Sikhs totally reject the caste system of the Hindus, however, believing that everyone has equal standing in the eyes of God.

Sikhism is strongly non-elitist and it is customary in its temples to sit on the floor to emphasize that everyone is of equal value. Many Sikhs follow the teachings of living gurus. They pray many times a day and also worship in temples known as *gurdwaras*.

Bahá'i faith

Just as Christianity arose from Judaism, so the Bahá'i faith developed from Islam. It is now a worldwide faith with around six million followers. They believe that there is only one God, the source of all creation who is transcendent and basically unknowable. However, he has sent and continues to send great prophets to reveal the word of God. These prophets are considered to have been: Adam, Abraham, Moses, Krishna, Zoroaster, Buddha, Jesus Christ, Mohammad and the Báb.

'The Báb' was the title assumed by Siyyid Ali-Muhammad (1819–50 CE), who lived in Persia. It means 'the gate' and, on 23 May 1844 (considered the founding of the faith), he explained that the purpose of his mission was to herald the arrival of 'One greater than Himself', who would fulfil the expectations of all the great religions. His followers became known as Babis and many were martyred for their beliefs in the religious unrest that followed. The Báb was executed in 1850, as he was seen as a threat to orthodox Islam.

The Manifestation predicted by the Báb was one of his followers, who became known as Bahá'u'llah and spent the last 40 years of his life in prison or exile. His son Abdu'l-Bahá became leader after his death.

The Bahá'i believe in the unity of all the great world religions – not that they are identical, but that they have all sprung from the same source. They assert that every person has an immortal soul, which, at death, passes to the spirit world – 'a timeless and placeless extension of our own universe'.

Prayer and fasting are a strong part of the faith; work is regarded as a form of worship and holy days are observed. Members of the faith also make at least one pilgrimage to the Shrine of the Báb and the houses in which Bahá'u'llah lived. They believe that unity is the key to peace and that eventually the world will be ruled by one single government, led by Bahá'is. Principles of freedom of speech, equality and tolerance are strongly promoted and they believe in scientific enquiry guided by spiritual principles. However, this tolerance is not extended to homosexuality, and women are excluded from serving in the Universal House of Justice, its highest religious court.

Vodun or voodoo

This grouping includes related religions such as Candomble, Macumba, Santeria, Lucumi and Yoruba.

A variety of religions with shared concepts and beliefs can be traced back to the West African Yoruba people. When the Yoruba were forced into slavery, they took their religion to Haiti and other Caribbean islands. The word *Vodun* equates to an African word for 'spirit'. Very similar religions (Umbanda, Quimbanda and Candomble) can be found in South America.

There are an estimated 60 million people practising Vodun worldwide. Each group follows a slightly different spiritual path and worships a slightly different pantheon of spirits, which are known as Loa. Traditional belief includes a chief god, Olorun, who is remote and unknowable. He authorized a lesser god, Obatala, to create the world and all life in it. However, these two gods had a battle that led to Obatala's temporary banishment. There are also hundreds of lesser gods and spirits, including Erzulia, goddess of love; Erinle, spirit of the forests; Ogou Balanjo, spirit of healing; Ogun, spirit of war; Baron Samedi, spirit of the graveyard; Agwe, spirit of the sea; Sango, spirit of storms; and Osun, spirit of healing streams. Many Loa are similar to Christian saints, in that they were once people who led exceptional lives. Vodun has many other features in common with Roman Catholicism and, indeed, in the past many slaves worshipped the Loa under the guise of Christianity.

Vodun ceremonies aim to make contact with the spirits and gain their help and favour by the offering of gifts and animal sacrifices. These ceremonies are elaborate, consisting of a feast prior to the main ritual; creation of a *veve* (a pattern of flour or cornmeal on the floor – each Loa has a particular pattern); chanting, rattling and drumming; and dancing by the priest (called a *houngan* or *mambo*) and the students (*hounsis*) until someone becomes possessed by a Loa and falls. The possessed dancer will be treated with great respect and takes on the characteristics of the Loa. An animal is usually sacrificed – its blood feeds the Loa. It is normally then cooked and eaten.

Followers of Vodun believe that each person has a soul composed of two parts: a *gros bon ange* (literally, 'large good angel') and a *ti bon ange* (or 'little good angel'). The *ti bon ange* leaves the body during sleep and when a person is possessed by a Loa during a ritual. These are dangerous times, when the *ti bon ange* can be damaged or captured by evil sorcery while free of the body (this corresponds to the belief in the astral body).

Vodun is a much misunderstood religion, mainly through the efforts of Hollywood! It conjures images of zombies, human sacrifice, graveyard rituals, murderous curses, necromancy and black magic. Certainly, it is fair to say that some hougans do engage in sorcery and a few mix both good and bad magic, but generally magic is used to bring healing and good fortune. Zombies, meanwhile, are considered to be people under the influence of powerful drugs, with no will of their own. As for the classic 'voodoo dolls' of horror movies, they are not commonly used; only occasionally in South America are they employed as a means of cursing.

Pagan religious traditions

The terms *pagan* and *neo-pagan* refer to a collection of separate religions which share common themes. These include Wicca and witchcraft, paganism and heathenism, shamanism, druidism, Asatru (Norse paganism), goddess worship and re-creations of ancient religious traditions such as the Celtic, Egyptian, Greek, Roman, Sumerian and Norse (among others).

These systems of belief were all persecuted in the past and, in many cases, little remains of the original practice and tradition. Modern followers have had to reconstruct their religions from ancient sources of information. Some have used channelling (obtaining information from the spirit realm) or intuition to fill the gaps.

Even today, these groups face much misunderstanding and persecution. Christianity, in particular, has confused the pagan faiths with Satanism (which has nothing to do with paganism and is, in fact, an offshoot of Christianity).

All pagans worship and revere nature. There is a deep reverence for the life force and the cycles of life and death within nature. Pagans celebrate a wheel of seasonal rituals which, while having deep spiritual meanings, are also an excuse for festivity and socializing.

Paganism puts great emphasis on individual responsibility and integrity. The classic pagan tenet is 'Do what thou wilt, but harm none' – which is often woefully misunderstood. It means that every individual has the duty to discover his or her Self and to develop it as fully as possible, in harmony with the outer world. We can do whatever we feel it requires to fulfil this, providing we do not hurt anyone else. Most pagans venerate both female and male principles of life – the Goddess and the God.

The pagan path is becoming very popular. People are drawn to the flexibility of this spiritual tradition (you can practise it in small groups or on your own). It is also very much in tune with present-day thoughts and concerns (the environment, balance between the sexes, self-development, interest in ritual and ceremony). Most pagans also believe that fun and laughter should be an essential component.

14 Prayer

In the past, prayer was as essential a part of everyday life as meals. As a child, I was taught to pray and indeed prayed in a very formulaic way for close on 25 years. But, nowadays, few people, apart from those with standard religious beliefs, actually pray.

This is a shame, as prayer is a very simple, yet immensely comforting, piece of soul work. It is 'talking' to God, Goddess or whatever it might be that is larger and knows more than us. Prayer means setting aside a time to unload our worries, our concerns and our anxieties – and also to share our joys, our triumphs and our gratitude.

Prayer is an intrinsic part of many religions: Christians pray to God, Christ and (in the Roman Catholic tradition) to Mary, Mother of God. Muslims turn towards Mecca and prostrate themselves in prayer. Hindus pray to the numerous deities of the Hindu pantheon. Wiccans pray to the Goddess, pagans to Mother Earth. A prayer can be as simple as 'Thank you, God,' or 'Please protect me and keep me safe', or it can be an elaborate series of words which form a traditional prayer. By ignoring or dismissing prayer, we just may be missing out on something deeply important. Psychologist and theologian Dr Walter Weston certainly thinks so. He has spent years researching the science of prayer and shares some remarkable findings in his book *How Prayer Heals*. 'The evidence indicates that humans accumulate, attune, focus and transmit an energy that heals,' he writes.

Recently, research has shown that prayer can significantly help AIDS patients. A study by the American Psychosomatic Society in Florida divided 40 equally ill patients into two groups. The group receiving prayer did not know that volunteers from ten religions and healing traditions were praying for them for an hour a day for a week. After 6 months, the group who had been prayed for had spent an average of 10 days in hospital compared to 68 days for the control group. Those receiving prayer also reported a decrease in emotional distress.

What does prayer mean to you?

Many of us recoil from the idea of prayer because of bad childhood experiences. Prayer might conjure up feelings of kneeling for long, boring periods, hands clasped, until your knees are sore. Or it might be associated with dreary visits to church, synagogue, mosque or temple. Take a few moments to think about what prayer means to you.

- When you think about praying, what images and sensations come to mind?
- What feelings and emotions emerge? Some of us will find resentment towards parents lies under the surface, or dislike of a priest or religious leader. I can remember feeling angry as a child that people in the church were hypocrites, gossiping cruelly after the service.
- Did you enjoy praying or dislike it? What did you like or dislike? Often it's the form of prayer that is the problem.

Mantras – a different form of prayer

Many people now commonly use mantras as a form of prayer and meditation. A mantra is simply a word or phrase used repetitively to enter a state of prayer and awareness of God. It can be just one word, such as 'ohm', or a series of words, such as the Hari Krishna chant.

Muslims repeat the name of Allah or the other Names of God; Quabalists tone the G-d-names; Tibetan Buddhists turn the prayer wheel chanting 'Aum mani padme hum', while Catholics recite the rosary while fingering rosary beads and Hindus repeat a mantra as they pass each bead of the mala through their fingers.

Finding the kind of prayer that works for you

There is no 'right' way to pray. You have to find what works for you. The following are just suggestions, nothing more.
- Some people will feel drawn to rediscover some of the beautiful old melodic prayers of traditional religion. You may want to move outside your childhood, or best known faith, and explore other traditions – perhaps the poetical Sufi tradition, or a Quabalistic prayer, or the prayers of the early Christian mystics, or even non-denominational New Age-type prayers.
- You may wish to make up your own prayers – or find pieces of poetry or prose that have meaning for you. Of course, you do not need to have a proper 'format' – many people simply talk to God, as if He/She/It were another human being. If you find it hard to talk to someone in your head, use the Gestalt empty-chair technique (page 26) and imagine God is sitting on the chair opposite you.
- You may wish to chant a mantra or try toning sounds.
- Some people find the best prayer is silence. Simply sit, kneel, stand or lie, and still your mind.
- Gazing at a religious object, painting or symbol can often become a form of prayer. It need not be a purpose-made artefact – it could be a stone, a piece of wood, a shell or a beautiful view or corner of nature. Some people pray leaning against a tree, or gazing into a fire or pool.

Hints on praying

If you're really stuck, think about the following:
- God, or the Higher Power, loves you unconditionally. Nothing that you say will shock. He or She will simply be delighted to hear from you!
- Don't worry about what words you use or don't use. It is your intention that matters, not how clever your vocabulary is.
- Use your prayer time as an opportunity to be totally honest, totally yourself. Share every part of your life – good and bad. Prayer isn't necessarily about just spiritual matters – God will be as interested in your exam worries or your insomnia as your quest for inner knowing and piousness!
- Be prepared for your prayers to be answered – though not always in the way you expect. Prayer can be very powerful.

15 Sacred Space

How do you feel when you walk into a church or temple? There is usually a sense of peace, an indefinable sense of walking into somewhere sacred, holy. It is what the Greeks called *tenemos*, a sanctuary. We all need places where we can feel safe and secure, peaceful and protected – on a daily basis. These need not be anywhere as grand as a synagogue or mosque – we can find peace within our own four walls.

When we walk through our front doors, we should be able to leave the stresses and strains of the outside world behind. A home should provide us with a sanctuary for the soul, a haven for the senses. It should be an oasis of calm and security, a place where we can be totally ourselves.

Think about how you feel when you walk into your home. Does a wonderful sense of peace and happiness descend on you, or do you feel irritated and stressed the moment you step through the door? If your house is a true haven, you will feel full of wellbeing – able to relax completely when needs be; energized and vitalized when that's the order of the day. If you constantly feel depressed, jumpy, nervous or just plain exhausted in your home, it is not serving your soul needs.

Why should our homes be so very important? I believe it's because a home is a symbol of the world; it represents our own mini-world, our own Mother Earth. When we feel safe and comfortable in our homes, we feel more able to deal with the often frightening outside world. Deep in our psyches, we recognize that a house or apartment is far more than a mere structure: our home is not just a place where we can keep out of the elements; it's far more than merely somewhere to eat and sleep.

What do you need from your home?

We are all different. Your ideal home may be a country cottage or cabin, simple and full of rustic charm. For someone else, the perfect place is an inner-city loft, vibrating to the constant hum of humanity. It could be a one-room apartment or a huge mansion. Before we set out to make our homes sacred, we must discover exactly what we need from them. There are many ways to find the elements of your perfect home. Try these:

- What kinds of home did you live in as a child? Think back. What did you like about them? Are there any elements of those homes that fill you with nostalgia?
- Let your mind wander over the places you loved when you stayed in them. Maybe a certain holiday cottage? A hotel or retreat? What did they have in common? Often this will not be the physical structure of the place, but a feeling. Try to pinpoint that feeling and figure out ways by which you might reproduce it in your home.

- Get out some paints and paper, and try painting an image of your soul home. It need not be an actual representation – it could be a series of colours or shapes. Don't think too much about it, just paint and see what happens. You might like to try painting with your non-dominant hand or with your eyes shut. Then sit back and see what your intuition says about the images you have created.
- Take out a pile of magazines and make a treasure map. Look for images that spell 'home' to you. You may be surprised at what your unconscious craves. Cut out the pictures and make a montage on a large sheet of paper. Place it somewhere you will notice it throughout the day – you can add or take off images as you see fit. It doesn't matter if the homes are out of your price range or beyond possibility – you are looking for the elements. You may not even choose pictures of homes or interiors – they could be pictures of people looking calm, families enjoying themselves or just colours or impressions. It's a kind of esoteric wish list.

Making a soul home

Once you know what you need from your space, you can start to make it a healing home, a soul home. A soul home is certainly not a place of clutter and chaos, but equally it is not a show home. Investing your home with soul is not about spending a fortune on new furniture and interior designers: it's about making your home a refuge for the senses, a retreat for the spirit. Some houses make you feel uncomfortable the moment you walk in. They look beautiful, but you hardly dare sit down in case you crease the cushions. You worry that your children might make a mess or your dog put pawprints all over the carpet. This kind of house is a statement – like the latest designer clothes or the smartest sports car. Hollow. The ideal soul home is nothing like that: it should be an oasis of delight and refreshment. How your home looks is important, but it also needs to feel good. Where possible, choose softly rounded shapes – in feng shui terms, soft contours help good energy to flow. In human terms, we tend to feel more comfortable nestled in a generous sofa with plump cushions than perched on a stiff, square chair. Think about sense-friendly textures, too. Given the choice between a luxuriously sensuous sheepskin rug and a scratchy, itchy synthetic rug, on which would you prefer to stretch out? Choose natural fabrics and furnishings as much as possible – they connect us with the natural world and make us feel more at home.

Do-it-yourself home protection

It's one thing adding texture and comfort to your home, but how do you bring in the right atmosphere and mood? Many of the techniques in this book (particularly the space-cleansing techniques on pages 97–8) will help, but you can start by trying this very simple ritual, a version of which exists in virtually every ancient culture:

1 Stand in the centre of your home and spend a few moments simply centring yourself. Close your eyes and gently follow your breathing. Feel the tension dropping away from your body and mind.

2 Now visualize a small glowing point of light deep in your heart. It shines with a clear, pure, bright white light.

3 Expand the point of light so that it becomes a bubble of light, one that surrounds your entire body. You know that, within this bubble, you are safe and protected, serene and secure.

4 Now take the bubble out even further, so that it encompasses your entire house or apartment, cocooning it in healing, transformative light. Imagine the protective bubble removing any negativity from your home, leaving it a pure, beautiful place of safety and serenity.

5 Gradually come back to normal awareness, armed with the knowledge that you have started to transform your home.

The elements

One of the nicest, and easiest, ways to bring a sense of magic and joy into your space is to ensure you have all the elements represented. This gives a home balance. Most people tend to favour one or two elements, and you can often tell which they are by the look and feel of their homes. For example, fiery people will generally be drawn to strong, vibrant, powerful colours, while watery people will tend to gravitate towards artistic homes full of paint effects and often piled high with clutter! Air homes are typically clean, airy (of course!) and spacious, and tend towards minimalism. Earthy homes will have lots of wood and stone, and natural colours such as greens, browns, taupes and russet – autumnal (fall) hues.

If you can, try to introduce all four elements. Here are some suggestions.

EARTH Earth grounds us, gives us safety, stability and a centre. It often represents the physical, our bodies and the earth itself.
- The most obvious way of bringing earth into your home is with natural stone and rock.
- Salt, too, represents earth and can be very useful in rituals and cleansings. Natural sea salt is best.
- Crystals are powerful storehouses of earth energy. Visit a crystal store and let your intuition pick the stone 'meant' for you. You could dedicate a crystal as your 'house' stone, or even have one for each room. For example, a rose quartz is a lovely protective stone for a child's bedroom.

WATER Water soothes and calms, and it is purifying and healing. It often represents our emotions.
- Install an interior waterfall – it's soothing and also very good feng shui (see pages 42–3).
- Bowls of water – perhaps with added flowers or petals – bring the element of water into the home and also provide valuable humidity.
- Introduce water into rituals by spraying rooms with a plant mister – you can add flower remedies (see pages 69–71) or aromatherapy oils if you wish, to intensify the beneficial effect.

AIR Air is invigorating, fresh and incisive. It often represents the intellect, the sharp power of the mind.
- Incense, smudging (see pages 98–9) and burning aromatherapy oils all attract the spirits of the air and can be used in ritual (see Chapter 16).
- Open your windows once or twice a day and let the fresh breeze blow through your home.

FIRE: Fire is pure energy – it ushers in new possibilities and is also protective. Fire often represents the will and the energy of the heart.

- Candles can be used both in rituals and to energize your home. But make sure they're safe (placing them in a bowl of sand or water is a good idea – and keep them well away from children and animals).
- An open fire is a comforting place beside which to meditate and dream.

Space cleansing

Space cleansing is one of the simplest yet most effective ways of shifting your home's atmosphere. It's an intrinsic part of most ancient cultures, yet here in the West it's a forgotten art. Vestiges of it remain in the wafting of incense around a church; the bells ringing out are a form of sound cleansing, purifying the parish.

Imagine how your house would be if you hadn't physically cleansed it for ten years? Not a pleasant thought. Yet few houses have ever been spiritually cleansed and so they become full of stagnant energy, old atmospheres and stuck emotions.

That may sound strange, but think about this. How often have you walked into a room and thought you could 'cut the air with a knife'? You are picking up the heavy emotional energy left by an argument or row. How often have you walked into a place and thought: 'I don't like the feeling of this place'? Or, conversely, walked in and thought: 'Oh, this is nice. I feel at home'? You are picking up on the 'atmosphere', the layers of emotional energy that have attached to the walls of the place.

Cleansing your home on an energy level is one of the most important things you can do to make it really your home, rather than the repository of the feelings, emotions and 'stuff' of its previous inhabitants.

Clearing clutter

Before you can start the esoteric work, you need to clear the clutter that invariably accumulates in every home. You don't have to get rid of everything, turning your home into a minimalist showpiece, but you do need to clear out the mess so that you can focus on what is important in your life. See the section on clutter on pages 40–1.

Remember that mess and clutter affect us on three different levels. Physically, clutter attracts dust and dirt, so a messy house will be a nightmare for anyone who suffers from allergies. You can never properly clean a messy house – and cleanliness is next to soulfulness! Psychologically, clutter makes us feel irritable and tense. Piles of disorganized letters and bills; rooms stuffed with objects; newspapers, magazines and toys lying everywhere all make us feel anxious – our subconscious knows there is work to be done and worries. Finally, on an energy level, clutter is a nightmare, as qi, or subtle energy, cannot flow smoothly and easily. It becomes stuck and turns stagnant, affecting our health and wellbeing. If you still find this process hard, think about what the Chinese sages said: when you clear away your clutter, you are making room for something new and exciting to come into your life.

How to space cleanse

1 Take a bath or shower. You might like to add a couple of drops of rosemary oil, which helps to purify your aura. Dress in clean, comfortable clothes, but keep your feet bare and remove all jewellery and your watch.
2 Go to the centre of your home and spend a few moments with your eyes shut, quietly breathing and centring yourself. You may be able to contact the spirit of

your house and ask for its help. If you have any religious beliefs, you may like to ask for help in whatever way feels right to you.

3 Start to 'clap out' your home. Move slowly and steadily around your home, clapping in every corner. Clap your hands, starting at the bottom of the wall and swiftly clapping on up towards the ceiling, as high as you can. You may need to repeat this several times in each spot – until the sound of your clapping becomes clear. As you clap, visualize your clapping dispersing any stagnant energy.

4 When you have finished clapping, wash your hands.

5 Go around your home balancing the energy with a bell or a rattle. Imagine the sound clearing any last vestiges of old energy.

6 Return to the centre of your space and once more close your eyes and breathe. How does your home feel now? Can you detect the difference?

7 Stamp your feet to ground yourself and have a good shake and stretch. It's also a good idea to have something to eat and drink after this ritual.

Note: do not perform space cleansing if you are unwell, pregnant or menstruating, or if you feel nervous or apprehensive.

Smudging

Smudging is the common name given to the Sacred Smoke Bowl Blessing, a powerful cleansing technique from the Native American tradition. Smudging calls on the spirits of sacred plants to drive away negative energies and put you back into a state of balance. It is the psychic equivalent of washing your hands before eating and is used as an essential preliminary to almost all Native American ceremonies. Smudging can be used to cleanse yourself before any form of ritual work or space cleansing. Before you undertake any form of ritual work, you should smudge the items you will be using (such as crystals, bowls of water, salt, candles, etc.). Smudging can also be used as a form of space cleansing in itself.

Do-it-yourself smudging

Smudge sticks are available in most New Age shops (commonly made from sagebrush, cedar and/or sweetgrass).

1 Light the end of your smudge stick and let it burn for a few minutes until the tip starts to smoulder.

2 Take off your shoes and remove any jewellery. Stand in a relaxed posture.

3 Feel the earth solid beneath your feet and ask Mother Earth to keep your feet solidly and safely on the ground.

4 Feel your head lifting up towards the sky and ask Father Sky to remind you of your link to Spirit. Remember you stand between the earth and the sky, balanced.

5 Now waft the smoke towards your heart. Hold the smudge stick away from you and use a feather to waft the smoke towards you, then take the smudge smoke over your head, down your arms and down the front of your body. Imagine the smoke lifting away all your negative thoughts, emotions and energies.

6 Breathe in the smudge, visualizing the smoke purifying your body from the inside. (Note: be careful if you suffer from asthma or respiratory difficulties.)

7 Bring the smoke down the back of your body to the ground. Visualize the last vestiges of negativity being taken back into the earth and away into the air.

8 Next, ask the spirits of the herbs to replace any negativity with pure, positive energy. Imagine you are surrounded by gentle, loving energy. Breathe in positivity, courage and love.

9 Thank the smudge stick, then put it out by dowsing it in earth or sand.

Shrines and altars

People have built altars and shrines for thousands of years. Archaeologists have found evidence of primitive altars, sacred objects and figurines all over the world: building altars is a very deep-seated human urge.

Altars have taken many shapes and forms. The first were probably the natural sacred spaces: places that seemed to our ancestors heavily imbued with the sacred; perhaps the dwelling place of a god, goddess or nature spirit. Mountain tops, caves, springs and groves were freely venerated. Offerings would be left and, over time, the place would become a natural shrine. As humans learnt more sophisticated building techniques, they used their architecture to create temples, churches and mosques as homes for Spirit.

Throughout history, the simpler tradition of home altars and shrines has endured. Many religions have continued the practice unbroken to the present day: step into any orthodox Hindu or Roman Catholic home and you will usually find a shrine. Images of Buddha and Kuan Lin will adorn the homes of a Buddhist or Taoist. For Native Americans, the medicine wheel is a gateway to Spirit, while most modern Wiccans have one or more altars with images of the Goddess and nature.

Personal altars can serve many purposes. Above all, they offer us the chance to make the Divine personal – an altar should always reflect our personality, our beliefs, our needs. Everything you place on your altar should have meaning. That way, whenever you see your altar, you become mindful of the sacred in your life.

Equally, you can make altars for specific purposes – to bring more of a certain energy into your life. Altars serve to concentrate our intentions. So, if you want to bring more success, or love, or peace into your life, you could construct an altar specifically geared to that purpose.

Candles

There are many varying associations for the different colours, but I find these work well:

BLUE For meditation or bedroom altars where you want to relax and be soothed.

PURPLE For psychic development or spiritual awareness. Purple is good for a private meditation altar.

GREEN For a healing altar, to bring balance, peace and harmony. Green can also be used in rituals to attract wealth or abundance.

YELLOW For friendship and joyful altars; use also when you want to increase your communication, good luck and wisdom. This is a good colour for a home-office altar or for a teenager facing exams.

RED For passion and energy. Red is good for attracting romance and sex.

PINK For when you are seeking love or wanting to conceive a child.

Building a home altar

Every home should ideally have a central 'home' altar that holds the spirit of the house and offers refuge and a home for the sacred. You may automatically know where it should be – maybe there is already a sort of subconscious altar there. If not, close your eyes and centre yourself, breathing calmly. Ask for guidance on where to place your altar – from your higher self, from your guardians, from the spirit of your home. You will most likely find that you suddenly get a strong feeling or a vague sense of where your house altar should be.

However, you don't have to stop at just one altar – you can build them all over your home. Many ancient cultures have some kind of shrine or sanctuary on or around the threshold of the house, offering protection and signalling the shift from the outside world into the sacred home. A kitchen is a natural place for a homely altar offering thanks for all your blessings. A living room could be home to a family or friends altar, celebrating love and warmth. More private altars can be sited in your bedroom, study and meditation space. Even small spaces – such as window ledges, the top of a cupboard or a series of hanging baskets in your bathroom – can make effective homes for altars.

There are no set rules as to what you should put on your altar. Simply follow your intuition and be guided by what feels right. However, if you feel uncertain, there are various tried and tested formulae that will start you on the right track. Let's look at how to build a basic home altar.

The fundamental ingredients include candles, a bowl of water, an incense holder or aromatherapy burner, matches and a bowl of salt. Optional extras for your altar could include a healthy plant or vase of fresh flowers, favourite photographs, crystals, representations of divinities, natural objects (such as stones, wood or shells) and other meaningful objects.

The first items on the list represent the four elements, which are traditionally represented on any altar for balance and connection. Place them as you see fit. You may like to add flowers or petals to the water in your bowl. Choose an incense or aromatherapy oil that you like or which suits your purpose for your altar. The colour of the candle you choose may also reflect your purpose (see page 99).

Now add any items to personalize your altar. If you are building a home altar, it is customary to include pictures of members of your family or items made by them. Things that represent your common or various interests can be included, too. If you have a favourite deity, it is good to include an image or symbol: a figure of Buddha or the Goddess, a cross or Star of David, etc.

Feel free to play around with the arrangement until it feels right. Light your candle and let your mind wander over the altar. Does it provide a focus for meditation? Does it set your mind on interesting pathways? If so, it is doing its job.

Once you have grasped the basic principles of altar building, you will find it simple to create altars for any room or any purpose. Just bear in mind that you are providing a visual focus for your intent, so include items that have particular meaning and resonance for you.

Seasonal altars

Later in this section, we will be looking at how to get back in tune with the natural world, with the shifting rhythms of the seasons. One lovely way to start this process is to build seasonal altars – to mark the shift from one season to the next and to help you prepare for the lessons of that time.

WINTER SOLSTICE (YULE) 21 December: This date marks the Celtic Christmas and is a great family festival. It is a time to focus on the people we need, rather than the people we like! It is also a time to recognize that conflict has a place in life and that we must learn how to deal with it. A time to focus and to reflect, this is when we should gather our intent for the year to come. Most of us subconsciously make a Yule altar in the form of a Christmas tree or a mantelpiece arrangement, but it is also good to think consciously about it. Traditional colours are red and green. Consider including:

- Evergreens such as holly, mistletoe and ivy
- Bells and brightly coloured baubles
- Photographs of people who can't be with you at Yuletide
- Sweets and candy, mince pies, spices such as ginger or cinnamon, oranges (perhaps made into pomanders by sticking cloves in them in pretty patterns)
- A glass of wine, sherry or punch
- Candles in brightly coloured bowls
- Your resolutions for the year to come

SPRING EQUINOX 21 March: Marking the first day of spring, this festival ties in neatly with Easter for Christians and celebrates the return of life. It's a time for spring cleaning (both physically and emotionally); a time to get rid of whatever has stuck to you over the winter – both things and people you have outgrown. It's an expansive time – to reach out for what you need to move forwards in life. Construct a joyous, colourful altar, maybe covered with a clear green cloth. Think about including the following:

- Spring flowers, buds and branches of pussy willow
- Eggs – either natural or painted or dyed
- Hares, which are the traditional animals associated with the spring equinox, but you can also include the Easter bunny and chicks, or any young animals
- Hot-cross buns
- Images of the Goddess, who returns after her winter descent underground, or Christ on the cross, who died and was reborn
- Green and yellow candles
- Seeds (you could plant them afterwards – something nice to do if you have children, or even if you don't!)

SUMMER SOLSTICE (MIDSUMMER'S EVE) 21 June: This is the peak of the expansive energy of the year and the summation of what you are and have become during this upward surge of the year's energy. It's a time to gather together in large groups. This is an outward, sociable festival, a time to learn about your place in society and the world. It is a time to examine what you want from life and to look at who you really are. It's often celebrated as a big party! Let your altar reflect this:

- Predominantly red – a red cloth and red candles
- Lots of summer fruits and berries
- Heaps of summer flowers – the more colourful and profuse, the better
- If possible, magical midsummer herbs such as St John's wort, mugwort, vervain and thyme
- Pictures of friends and joyous party images

AUTUMN (FALL) EQUINOX 21 September: This is a new phase as winter starts to draw closer. The Earth Goddess has departed into the earth and the leaves are turning. It's a time for purification, for quiet, inward work when we stop to adjust ourselves to a less outdoor part of the year. It's a time for long-term planning, for letting go of parts of ourselves that no longer serve our essential being. It's a time to reconcile the opposites within us – looking at male and female, dark and light, young and old. Your altar should reflect this:

- Rich, russet autumn (fall) colours – deep reds, rusty yellows, dark greens, burnt oranges for your cloth and candles
- Wreaths of oak leaves and nuts
- Pumpkins, squash, apples and other fruits of the harvest
- Pine cones, nut kernels and dried herbs
- Coloured yarns, beads or shells – you could make necklaces, weaving in symbols of what you want from life
- Muslin herb bags (afterwards, place them in drawers to deter moths or use as bath bags)
- Opposing pairs of things – two stones, one black and one white; something rough and something smooth; something old and something new

16 Ritual

Rituals occupy a strange place in modern society. We either love all the paraphernalia they entail or hate the disruption they bring. Some people look forward to gatherings such as Christmas as a time of family, friends and fun; others feel horror as the first Christmas cards appear in the stores, dreading a season of stress and strain. Almost all of us, however, whatever our thoughts, go through the motions. Aside from stoically battling with Christmas, we dutifully bake birthday cakes and we don our best clothes to go to weddings, Bar Mitzvahs and funerals. Some of us even still make it to the traditional celebration of Harvest Festival.

Many people would say, in fact, that we have far too much ritual in our lives. Isn't life busy enough without having more plans to make, more occasions to celebrate? Compared to our forebears, however, we are seriously lacking in rituals. Ritual might seem outmoded, even unnecessary, but many experts insist that, in order to lead balanced, healthy lives, we need much more ritual, not less. Many psychotherapists believe that rituals – and plenty of them – should make up a central part of our lives.

We're not talking about dispatching a bunch of flowers for Mother's Day, a card for Father's Day or snatching a last-minute box of chocolates for Valentine's Day. For rituals to be healing and life-enhancing, they have to be more than duty – they have to have meaning. We don't need more commercial trappings; we don't need bigger and better Christmases: we simply need more personalized ones. Do you find yourself following exactly the same pattern every year at Christmas? Do you look forward to it or does its approach fill you with a sense of burden and horror at its commercialization? Are your rituals too rigid? Have they stayed the same over the years despite obvious changes in family members' ages or beliefs? If a ritual no longer works for you, you need to change it. Rituals should grow and evolve all the time.

An example might be reinventing a ritual to celebrate an anniversary. You might go out together or cook a special meal at home. You could give gifts that symbolize the past year you have spent together – something really thoughtful that has meaning. You might then talk about what you both want for the next year of your life – you could use it as a time to make your lists (as discussed in Chapter 7).

On a much smaller note, you might decide to start every morning with a kiss and end every evening with a word that you want to symbolize the next day – even tiny things such as this are rituals and, what's more, powerful ones.

Ancient ceremonies

Rituals were a central part of life for our ancestors. In pagan times, each year that passed was marked with regular seasonal festivals in which all community members participated. Experts believe that these were not, as has been commonly assumed, an attempt to control nature, but rather a means of coming to terms with the shifting rhythms of the seasons. By following the ups and downs of the year, people got to grips with the cycles of their own lives, learning that there are times of great energy and joy alongside times of quiet introspection; times of birth and rebirth, but inevitably also times of sadness, loss and death. Perhaps it is a subconscious yearning for these lost or denigrated celebrations that has, in part, caused the rising interest in paganism and other native, earth-based religions, with their plethora of satisfying rituals and celebrations.

Shan, a therapist and pagan priestess who taught me so much about ritual, insists on the importance of seasonal rituals: 'The seasons of the year are less crucial to our modern lives, with imported food, heated houses and indoor work,' she says. 'But our bodies and emotions still go through their important changes, which we are foolish to ignore. They can greatly enrich our lives if we honour their primal wisdom.' She notes that, according to the pagan calendar, there are 8 festivals a year, about one every 6 weeks. 'That gives us about 5 to 6 weeks of workaday life, then a break for a holiday or celebration – an entirely pleasant and very healthy rhythm,' she adds.

Between these seasonal festivals, our forebears celebrated important life events – birth, adolescence, menstruation, marriage, menopause and death. A few rituals remain, but are often stifled or derisory. Think of the wedding where the heart of the ceremony has been lost amid the paraphernalia of video cameras and social one-upmanship. Or the practice of 'drive-through' funerals in which mourners 'pay their respects' by observing the deceased on a video screen and recording their presence on a computer. How can tapping on a computer keyboard release pent-up grief? Better, undoubtedly, an old-fashioned wake when everyone sinks a few drinks and spends a day surrounded by family and friends talking about the deceased, reminiscing and celebrating that life, letting the tears flow when necessary, but recalling all the happy times as well. Surely therein lies healing and a growing acceptance of loss?

Good rituals are essential to our emotional, psychological and spiritual health. In a time when many of us live far from our family and don't even know our neighbours, rituals not only help us on a personal basis, but also give us a small sense of community, a sense of who we are and where we fit in the scheme of life. Without rituals, we drift. Today, however, we lack these essential rituals and ceremonies.

Rituals really can help us with difficult transitions such as puberty, menstruation and menopause; painful situations, such as divorce, death and illness; and even crises such as burglary, accidents and assault. Psychotherapists since the days of Jung have recognized the power of symbols, of age-old archetypes, of emotive ritual to cleanse the psyche and free the emotions. Say you have just recovered from a serious illness or come out of hospital, why not burn or bury a symbol of that time? Ritually discard your no-longer-needed medicines, burn your hospital bracelet. Alternatively, write a declaration celebrating your newfound health and vitality. It's a way of signalling to your unconscious mind that you are now well. Even the most ridiculous-sounding rituals can be effective. One couple who were always fighting agreed upon a ritual in which they put symbols of their quarrel 'on ice' in the freezer. They signed a pact to say that they could only fight about the issue after they had thawed the symbols out.

If you follow meaningful rituals, you will weather the inevitable changes of life far more easily.

Bath rituals

Rituals do not need to be complex or elaborate, as we have seen. They can easily be part of everyday life, giving us a chance to stop and centre ourselves, even if only for a few minutes. One opportunity to introduce an element of ritual is our daily washing routine.

Water is extremely cleansing and purifying, so it makes sense to use your regular bath or shower as an excuse for some deep, powerful cleansing. The purifying shower below is the perfect way to start your day, making you feel positive and upbeat about the day ahead. The bath is ideal for shedding the trials and tribulations of a stressful day.

Purifying shower

Start your day with this invigorating shower, which will help you feel positive and confident about the day to come.

1   As you step into the shower, imagine you are stepping under the clean, pure waters of a beautiful waterfall in the wilderness. While you stand under the waters, visualize the magical water washing away any negativity, leaving you full of energy and vigour for the day to come.

2   Wash yourself with a sponge and some uplifting aromatherapy oils (citrus or pine fragrances work well).

3   Consciously let go of any worries, concerns or anxieties. Imagine they are being sloughed off you as the water cleanses your body. Breathe in deeply and believe that the day ahead will be positive and full of joy. Any problems are simply challenges which you will overcome with ease.

4   Step out of your shower and have a wonderful day!

Deep-cleansing bath

This deep-cleansing bath is ideal as a 'winding-down' ritual at the end of the day.

1   Light candles all around your bath. If you like, you can also light an oil burner and put in a few drops of your favourite aromatherapy oils – sandalwood, camomile, geranium, lavender and ylang ylang are all good choices.

2   Your bath should be pleasantly warm, but not too hot. Add three drops each of your chosen aromatherapy oils (mixed in a little milk) and agitate the water to disperse them.

3   As you undress, imagine that you are dumping all your problems with your clothes. Start to let go of the stress, strain and any negativity of the day.

4   Sprinkle some sea salt on a damp face cloth. Gently scrub your entire body with small, circular movements. Work from the extremities of your body towards your heart. Imagine the purifying power of the salt loosening all the psychic grime of the day. (Note: consult your doctor first if you have high blood pressure or heart disease and do not use salt if you have any irritated or broken skin.)

5   Relax in your bath and visualize the healing water gently drawing out all the negativity and unpleasantness of the day. Soak for at least 20 minutes.

6   As you step out of the bath, look back and see the water as containing all the anger, sorrow, frustration, etc. of the day. Bless it, then let it go.

7   Having followed this ritual, you should find that you now sleep well and wake refreshed.

Mealtime rituals

Bring ritual into your life by investing mealtimes with a sense of the sacred. All religions teach that food is a blessing from the Divine and should be treated with respect and gratitude. No Jewish, Christian, Hindu, Muslim or Buddhist family would dream of scoffing a meal without saying a blessing and giving thanks. In China, food is considered to be a physical link between humans and the Gods: beautifully prepared meals are given as a sacred offering on the family altars. Begin by considering the following questions.

- How do you eat? At table with family or friends? While working? On the run?
- What do you eat? Do you prepare your own food or do you buy ready-prepared processed food?
- Do you ever really taste your food?
- Are you mindful when you eat?

The simplest of rituals can turn even the humblest sandwich into a feast for the spirit. The principles of making mealtime sacred are very straightforward – and can easily be adapted to fit your circumstances and preferences. Preparing 'soul' food need not involve new recipes or expensive ingredients. Follow these simple principles to transform the food you eat.

- Take care when choosing food – pick the freshest, most local, seasonal, organic food you can find. If you eat meat, ensure that it has been farmed with care and consideration for the animals. Perhaps think about growing some of your own food – even if it's just a window box with herbs.
- Say a prayer or blessing before you start to cook or prepare your food. Hold your hands over your ingredients and thank them for giving their life for you. Visualize the journey of your ingredients – how they grew, who tended them, how they came to be on your table. Ask them to help nourish you and family members, friends or guests with love.
- Prepare your food with love and attention. Concentrate on the task at hand – look on it as sacred meditation. Try not to distract yourself by watching television or listening to the radio as you cook. Take time to notice the textures, scents and look of the food you are cooking. Avoid gadgets and processors where possible – hand-chopping brings you closer into contact with the food.
- Think of your cooking as sacred alchemy. Remember you are using all the elements in your cookery – the earth from which your raw ingredients came; water to cook in; air you add as you stir or beat; and the fire of your stove.
- As you cook, pour in your hopes and wishes for the people who will eat your food. Focus your intention as you chop, stir, mix and blend. Cookery is a kind of spell-making. If you add herbs and spices with their magical properties, you can increase the power.
- Lay your table with care – even the simplest meals can be made special by adding a small vase of flowers (a posy of wild flowers, buds or leaves is cheap but lovely) or perhaps a candle. You could also scatter petals or pine cones on the tablecloth. Don't eat in front of the television or on the run!
- Serve your meal so it looks inviting and appetizing. Choose colours which complement each other.
- Say grace or a blessing before eating.

- Eat your food mindfully. Smell the different fragrances before you start to eat. Notice how you choose your food – be aware of putting it on your fork and in your mouth. Don't just swallow – really taste the food, feel its texture. Make each mouthful mindful.
- If you are eating with others, allow time during your meal for conversation and a sense of community. Don't race off afterwards – sit and talk.
- Clean up with mindfulness and gratitude, too. Try adding a few drops of mandarin oil to your washing-up liquid to invigorate your senses.

Blessings and graces

Blessings and graces have been said for millennia in many cultures and saying them is a simple ritual that makes a mealtime special. Every religion has its own varieties and, in the past, most families would have their favoured wordings. Nowadays, however, we rarely say grace – unless we happen to be at a large, formal occasion. Yet saying grace gives us the chance to think about all the blessings we enjoy and to offer thanks. Take the opportunity to bring this small but important ritual back into your everyday life.

1 Before you eat as a group, you might like to light several small candles around the table. Each person then says a few words of thanks, expressing pleasure at being together to share a meal.

2 Think about the processes which brought this food to your table. You might, for example, pick up a loaf of bread and think about the miraculous way it has come to you. It starts with a tiny seed which grows under the sun, nourished by the earth. It is harvested, threshed, milled into flour and then kneaded and baked into bread to feed you. Give everyone a piece of bread and invite them to give thanks in their own way for this gift of life.

3 Always try to be hospitable and welcoming to guests. Make some mealtimes special by inviting extended family, friends or neighbours. Is there someone needy who might appreciate an invitation – perhaps an elderly neighbour or someone who is new to the area and doesn't yet have friends who live close by?

4 Muslims often serve food in one large dish or on an immense platter. Everyone helps themselves from the same dish, choosing the portion of food closest to them. This symbolizes the sharing, caring aspect of the family or group – it draws people together. Try this, maybe by cooking something such as a large paella or experiment with Middle Eastern or African food, which lends itself well to this format.

5 Before you eat, pause a few moments for everyone to say their silent prayers of thanks and appreciation. Silent grace is a lovely idea, as it removes the need for what can become formulaic set graces and gives each person the chance to say whatever he or she wishes.

Family rituals

Think about rituals that could bind your family more closely. How could you make Christmas more meaningful? What would make a birthday more special? Think about the meaning behind any religious rituals you observe – don't simply go through the motions. In addition, think of other events that could be reasons for inspiring family rituals. The following might provide a starting point.

- **BIRTHDAYS** These are a pivotal point in the year. Try to make them meaningful and special – however old you are! You might want to think about all that has happened in the past year (maybe sharing it with your friends or family). Give thanks for everything good that happened and let go all the bad. Ask yourself what lessons you have learnt. Think about what you would like from the year to come. You might want to smudge yourself and consciously let go of any negativity (see page 98). Be aware that this is a new start for you, a new year full of fresh opportunities.

- **NEW YEAR** This is a traditional time for a fresh start. Perhaps you could gather the family together and burn some special incense or aromatherapy oil – something fresh such as lemon or bergamot. Each of you could make a list of what you most want from the coming year, first for yourself and then for your family as a whole. Take turns to share your visions. You might also work together preparing a special meal, putting all your hopes for the year to come in the pot.

- **A BIRTH** The birth of a baby is a miraculous event, one worthy of celebration. Alongside any traditional religious ceremony, you might do something small and personal for the family and close friends. You may want to call down protection from guardian angels, spirit animals or other deities on your child. You may want to introduce the baby to your community in some way – either with a gathering or simply by walking him or her around your neighbourhood in his or her buggy. Dedicating a crystal for the baby is a nice idea (rose quartz is especially appropriate). You might also take a leaf from the fairy tale of Sleeping Beauty and have everyone present offer the baby a 'gift' such as courage, joy or confidence.

- **HOLIDAYS** For most of us, getting ready for holidays can be a stressful time. Set aside a short space of time for everyone to gather and focus on what they want from the holiday. Light a candle and take it in turns to say what you need from your holiday and what you hope for. Think about activities you can do together (and pack the appropriate gear). Holidays are also an ideal opportunity to have time on your own for reflection, meditation or just vegging out with a good book, so agree beforehand how this will be achieved. Having clear, agreed expectations of each other will take away a lot of stress and irritation.

17 Nature

We have a strange relationship with nature. We seem to feel that we are separate from it, that nature is something to go and see as you might visit a zoo or a museum. Living in our centrally heated, air-conditioned houses, we barely need be aware of the changes in the weather, the passing seasons. Strolling around a supermarket for our food, we don't have to worry about how our crops are faring or whether there are animals to hunt to keep hunger at bay. If we get sick of the weather at home, we hop on a plane and go elsewhere, where the climate is more to our liking.

We want nature to be perfect and, when it doesn't behave as we want it to, we become irritated with it. We like to think we can control nature, to bend it to our will. We build our houses and factories where we wish; we tear down forests for development; we level mountains for roads or tunnel straight through them; and we pollute the seas, rivers, earth and air for the sake of modern, convenient chemicals.

Our ancestors would have been stunned by our attitude. They would have been terri-fied that the earth would retaliate – and maybe it has. For the truth is we cannot control nature, we cannot ever really 'rule' the earth. By trying to do so, we miss a vital soul lesson. Living in harmony with nature, accepting that we are no more and no less than another cog in the great wheel of life, is essential to our growth.

Some extreme ecologists say we need to get rid of our cars, abandon our houses and return to a life of hunter-gathering. We cannot, however, turn back the clock that far – it's impractical and a foolish pipe dream. We couldn't just drop our civilization like that, nor would most of us want to. It is possible to live more lightly on the earth, though, to stop interfering so grossly in its life, to prevent our egoism and greed from destroy-ing our only home.

Taking responsibility for the earth, for our home, is a crucial part of the work of the soul. We modern soul-seekers cannot be hermits, burying our heads in the sand. We are part of the world and have to take responsibility for it. If we want our children and our chil-dren's children to feel their souls fill with the majesty of an ancient forest, with the fluting call of a lark, we have to take a stand. Once again, it need only be small gestures, small beginnings – but we do need to take these steps. And taking steps like these, however small, gives us a sense that at least we're doing something. In a tiny way, it gives us back a little piece of personal power in what is an increasingly bureaucratic world.

How do you live on the earth?

Start to think about how you live on the earth. The earth is our only home – we physi-cally need it. Beyond this primal power, our souls require a world that still has the ability to move and awe us. If all we have left is a world of concrete, plastic and fast food, what is left to nourish our souls? Think about what you could do to help, in your own small way.

- Start recycling household waste – separating glass, cans, papers and plastics. Organic waste (except potato peelings and meat) can become rich compost if you have a garden. You don't need a huge space to compost – there are now smart, speedy, smell-free composters on the market, so use one. Composting also saves gardeners money on expensive soil improvers.
- Think about leaving the car at home on some days and walking or cycling to work instead. If possible, work out a car-share with colleagues or friends.
- Make a commitment to eating organic food that has not been grown with harmful pesticides, herbicides, fungicides and hormones.
- Buy secondhand furniture (remember, antiques are basically fifth-or-more-hand!) or at least choose furniture that comes from sustainable sources.
- Support campaigns for better public transport so that we need fewer new roads and developments.
- Donate money to environmental groups that are trying to save the world's rainforests and other precious resources.
- Write to politicians until they open their eyes and realize that, beyond of industry and growth, profit and vested interests, the environment must be our prime concern.

Exploring the elements

Few of us are really in touch with the elements. We tend to avoid them (keeping inside when it's raining or windy) or experience them in sanitized forms (such as swimming pools). These very simple exercises plug you in to elemental energy – they are especially important if you live in a city or built-up area.

STONE
Go to a place in nature (ideally wild, but, if not, a park or garden) and find 'your' stone, one that seems to speak to you in some way. Don't worry if you don't find it immediately (remember, patience is one of the key lessons of nature), and trust your intuition.

Pick up the stone and sit quietly with it. If it is too large, sit by it. Explore it with all your senses: really look at it, touch it, smell it. Now, perhaps hardest of all, listen to it. What has the stone seen in its long life? What lessons does it have for you? Imagine you are that stone. How does it feel to possess its energy? What would life be like as a stone? Where is your heart, your centre?

Spend some time each day meditating on stone. Think about the properties of stone that could be useful for you in your everyday life – and in your soul life.

WATER
Water feels so different from stone. You can't keep it and hold it, but you can explore it in its many different forms. If possible, spend some time by a spring or stream, investigating its exuberant energy. Once again, use all your senses. Think about its lessons. It's a fascinating process to follow a stream from its source to the place where it joins the sea if you can. Note the changes along the way. What parallels can you draw with your own life?

The ancients believed that every stream and river had its own spirits, the naiads: can you sense the spirit of the water? How would it appear?

Think about having a small water fountain in your home or outside in the garden. Use it as a place for contemplation and a chance to connect with the water spirit.

WOOD

Pick a tree and spend time observing it minutely. Look at its shape, how it grows, where it grows. Investigate its bark, roots, branches and leaves. Sit with your back against its trunk and quietly absorb its energy and share some of your own in return. Hugging is optional, but often irresistible (particularly if you are upset or confused). Employ all your senses and try to hear what the tree is saying. Again, every tree was believed to have a spirit, a dryad. What kind of spirit does your tree have? Can you talk to it? Compare the energy of different kinds of trees. Pick up a piece of dead wood and sense the difference to that of living trees.

Spend some time learning about trees so that you can then identify them and know their lore.

FIRE

If there is somewhere totally safe (with no chance of starting bush fires or causing damage), it can be inspiring to build and tend a small fire outdoors. Watch how a tiny spark glimmers into life. For a time it seems that it won't catch, but then it suddenly shoots away, crackling and sparking. Watch how the colours change in the flames, observe the shapes of the flames and see if you can see (or imagine) the salamanders, spirits of fire. See how hungrily the fire devours the wood, licking along its branches. Then, as the fire subsides, watch the embers glowing and, finally, the wood transforming into charcoal and ash. What would it be like to be fire? How would it feel?

Roast chestnuts or bake potatoes in the glowing embers as you reflect on the lessons of fire – how it can be so destructive yet also so helpful. Does its destructiveness have a purpose? Do we sometimes need to burn away our dross and start afresh? At home, light a candle to remind yourself of fire and its lessons.

AIR

Go to a high place – the top of a mountain, crest of a cliff or brow of a hill – to experience the element of air. Feel yourself on top of the world and breathe the fresh, clear and invigorating air deeply and fully. What would it be like to be the wind? How would it feel to be of air, able to enter any crack, however tiny? Imagine the air coming into your lungs, exchanging oxygen for carbon dioxide, then coming out again.

Next, go somewhere different – a low place, a forest, swamp or underground cave. How is the air different? Contrast it also to the air in a city, amid heavy traffic. What are we doing to our air?

It can be difficult to come to terms with air: we can't see it, we can barely feel it. Yet its lessons are important and it's worth trying to connect with this essential element. Remind yourself of air by lighting incense, burning aromatherapy oils or smudging, allowing the scent to rise on the air and up to the heavens.

Linking ourselves with nature

Few of us spend time in nature. Even if we consider ourselves 'outdoor' people, few of us actually stop long enough to look and listen in a meaningful way. Set aside some time to go to a wild place – ideally not a park, but somewhere where you can be alone. First of all, just sit on the grass (or sand or stone). If it's wet, do sit on a groundsheet, but otherwise let your body connect with the earth. Close your eyes and let your other senses take over. What do you hear? At first, you will notice only obvious sounds (birdsong, the wind, far-off mechanical sounds perhaps), but as your listening becomes more attuned you may hear other, tinier sounds. Try to spend at least 20 minutes like this. You may find it disorientating, even a little scary (if you aren't used to being out in nature), so perhaps have a friend near by.

If you feel comfortable, repeat the exercise lying down on the earth. Feel your limbs sink into the earth, feel the ground supporting your head, your whole body. Work through your body, consciously relaxing each part – from your feet right up to your head. Now bring your awareness to your solar plexus and feel it becoming soft and warm. Visualize a golden cord of shimmering energy linking your solar plexus with the heart of the earth, grounding you and rooting you. Slowly stand up and feel your feet rooted to the ground, anchored and safe. The connection with the earth rises up through the ground, through your feet and up your legs into your torso. It pauses a moment at your solar plexus, then rises up again, through your heart, your throat, your head, and bursts through and rises up to the sky. You feel yourself standing, solidly grounded with the earth beneath, yet linked to the sky above. Know that this is your place – safely held between the earth and the heavens.

Shamanism

While the so-called 'civilized' nations have mostly lost their relationship with nature, we can turn to those wise peoples who have kept alive the spirit of nature and the link between it and humankind. Many of the neo-pagan traditions (such as druidism, Wicca, etc.) forge a strong link with nature and believe it central to their way of life. These all have a strong shamanic element and, if we want to learn how to come back into balance with nature, we need to look to the shamans. Shamans exist all over the world, in places where the tradition has been kept alive. A shaman is basically someone who can walk and talk with the spirits and who has maintained a close link with nature. It's a form of spirituality that reveres the earth as a sentient, living, vibrant entity.

Shamanism is undergoing a huge surge in popularity – it's as if people recognize, at some level, that we desperately need the shamanic wisdom to put us back in touch with our souls and nature.

There isn't the space in a book this size to delve deeply into the myriad practices of shamanism, but we can take a look at some of the most important principles.

Medicine walking

In the shamanic view, there is no such thing as coincidence. Things happen because they are meant and because there is a lesson to be learnt. This can be seen in the broad picture of life – that sickness is a way for the body to insist on a much-needed rest; that losing a job might be a prelude to finding a better one; that the end of a relationship could be necessary for growth. But it can also be seen as a way of learning each and every day. Native Americans follow a practice known as the 'medicine walk', in which they go out into the wilderness and read, in every animal they see, every natural occurrence, a message. This can be a useful practice in everyday life. It helps us to become more aware of the natural world and also to appreciate that nature really can be our best teacher. Start to become aware of the world around you and ponder what messages it might have for you.

• What is the weather doing? What does it mean to you if it's raining, windy, snowing, hot and sunny? Think about your feelings and how they are reflected in the weather.

- What animals or birds do you see? Think about the associations any animals have for you personally. You might also like to look them up in books on symbolism or shamanic practice.
- What is the animal or bird doing? Is it behaving in a normal way or strangely? How does that resonate with you? Can you detect a lesson there? How are you like that animal in life, relationships, attitude?
- Pay attention to the plants, trees and flowers you see. Do any strike a particular chord? Perhaps a tree is growing in a curious way (does it remind you of anything?). Maybe there is a flower blooming in an unlikely place – what lesson does that have for you?
- If an animal crosses your path, it is particularly important. Spend some time meditating on that animal – or asking it what message it has for you.
- You don't have to be out in the country to medicine walk. There are messages on every city street as well. Be aware not just of the natural world, but also of the movement of buses, trains, people.

Spirit animals

Some animals have particular messages for you. Shamans believe that we all have special 'spirit animals' which can act as strong protectors and guides.
- Are there any animals which have always held a particular resonance for you? To which animals or birds are you drawn?
- Are there any animals or birds you really don't like? You may find you have a resistance because that particular animal has a tough lesson for you.
- Is there any animal you often dream about? If so, you could try getting in touch with it. When you next meet it in a dream, ask it whether it is 'your' animal (or you are 'its' human). If it agrees, you can ask it for advice or teaching.

In a similar way, you can take yourself into a deep meditative state (lie down and relax your body, then let your breathing become slow and regular). Imagine yourself in the kind of habitat your animal would inhabit (maybe a forest, a jungle, a mountain). Visualize it as clearly as you can and ask that, if the time is right, your spirit animal will come and meet you. If it does, again you should ask for its permission – and be willing to listen to any advice. Always be very respectful.

If you don't feel drawn to any animal in particular, you can still work with power animals. Perhaps the easiest way to do this is to start with the four great guardians of Native American belief. These are:
- **BEAR** Linked with the element of fire and the west, Bear's energy is strong, powerful and determined. Bear energy cleanses and gives energy.
- **EAGLE** Linked with the element of air and the east, Eagle's energy is inspirational, far-sighted and protective. Eagle energy clarifies.
- **BUFFALO** Linked with the element of earth and the north, Buffalo's energy is grounding and protective, and is said to give knowledge of life and death.
- **COYOTE** Linked with the element of water and the south, Coyote's energy is clever, quick-minded and swift. Coyote governs the emotions.

You can call on these powerful guardians for help at any time of need. Invoke Eagle when you need to keep your vision sharp and focused. Coyote can be very helpful in business meetings when you need to keep your wits about you. If you are in a situation when you feel uneasy or unsafe, Bear is a very comforting presence. Whenever you need some good, solid earthing, invoke Buffalo. Buffalo can also be a great friend if you cannot sleep – she ushers in sleep and bestows useful dreams.

Invoking the guardians

1 Stand with your feet planted firmly on the earth. Close your eyes and imagine a piece of string is gently pulling your head up towards the sky.
2 As you stand firmly between Mother Earth and Father Sky, you gradually become aware of four mighty creatures standing around you.
3 At your back, you feel the power of an enormous she-bear rearing up behind you, supremely protective. Nothing can harm you while Bear protects your back.
4 Before you, you feel the beat of powerful wings. A vast eagle, wings outstretched, turns and fixes you with its sharp, all-seeing eye. With Eagle's eyes ahead of you, you will be prepared for all eventualities.
5 On your right-hand side, you feel the warm breath of Buffalo. She is a comforting and calming figure, and will ground you and give you wisdom and forbearance.
6 As your left hand rests by your side, you feel rough fur under your fingers. It's Coyote, master of clever speech and swift evasive action. With Coyote at your side, you should always have a ready answer and be quick-witted and smart. But watch out: Coyote can be a trickster – don't rely on his honeyed tongue alone!
7 Spend some time with these great creatures, allowing their power to seep into your body and soul. Recognize that you can call on them whenever you need their strength. Thank them for introducing themselves to you, then come back to waking reality.

18 Retreating

Sometimes you don't just need a holiday, you need a retreat. In the past, going on retreat was an accepted part of life. Anyone with a religious turn of mind would simply take himself or herself off to a monastery or convent (or temple, sweat lodge or ashram) and spend some time in contemplation and prayer, often fasting and keeping silent throughout a period of vigil. It was a time to spend with God; a time to be quiet and hear the voice of your soul. It was a time to evaluate and reassess your life.

Retreating is enjoying a huge resurgence in popularity. There are retreats to suit every religious belief system and, if you are not particularly religious, there are secular or non-denominational retreats to suit every soul. Stafford Whiteaker, author of a guide to retreats, explains: 'A retreat is an inward exploration that lets your feelings open out, and gives you access to both the light and dark corners of your deepest feelings and relationships. It is simply the deliberate attempt to step outside ordinary life and relationships and take time to reflect, rest and be still. It is a concentrated time in which to experience yourself and your relationship to others and, if you are fortunate, to feel a sense of the eternal.'

What do you need from your retreat?

Before you decide on your retreat, take some time to ask yourself what you really want and need from your 'time out'.

- Do you want a structured retreat? Some offer a programme of features, such as prayer, meditation, visualization and lectures. Others will leave you to your own devices.
- Do you want to be with others or on your own? In many retreat centres, you can arrange to go at a very quiet time or have isolated accommodation. If solitude is important, you might consider arranging your own accommodation (e.g. a rented cottage). If you don't want to be alone, there are also many retreats where you can be part of the community.
- Do you want to follow a particular path or belief system? Retreats can be a perfect opportunity to investigate a religion and see what it offers you. Many religious retreats allow you to take part in community life to some extent (e.g. going to prayers or joining in communal meditation). Equally, others are not run according to any particular faith.
- Can you cope with the possibility of difficult feelings emerging? A lot of people find that the solitude and focus of a retreat can bring old or repressed emotions and memories to the fore. If you're not used to working with your emotions, it may be a good idea to choose a retreat that has skilled counsellors or wardens on hand.

- For how long do you want to retreat? If you're new to the concept, a weekend retreat might be the best option. Once you become used to the set-up, a week is usually the shortest recommended period. Some experienced retreaters will take themselves away for a month or even a year!

Food for retreating

Food can set the tenor for a good retreat. It really doesn't matter what you eat when you're retreating, but, for many people, diet is an important part of the mix. Whatever your choice, be mindful of your sustenance. Look back at the suggestions on cooking and eating mindfully on pages 106–7.

- You might think about a detoxifying retreat. Some people like to fast, but this should only be carried out under professional guidance. If you are in good health and the weather is warm, it's usually okay to try a juice fast of vegetable and fruit juices (but not for more than two days).
- Others see a retreat as a time for pampering and comfort: chocolate and a good bottle of wine might be the ticket.
- If self-catering, keep your food choices simple to prepare. You don't want to spend your entire retreat cooking! Often the most successful choices are easy soups, stews and casseroles (which can be prepared ahead and frozen), or salads, fruit, bread and cheese or cold meats.
- Always have plenty of fresh water. This could also be a good time to experiment with herbal teas or interesting juices. Have a large bowl of fresh fruit on hand for snacking.
- If you're planning to do a lot of exercise, make sure that you eat nutritious and satisfying food – think about some good protein choices.
- If you have problems related to food, be aware these may well intensify during a retreat. This isn't the time to go on a Draconian diet, but you may want to avoid the foods that you know 'block' your feelings – maybe bread, chocolate, sweets, etc. The same applies to alcohol.

What to do on retreat?

There are 101 different ways of retreating and it's entirely up to you to decide what you need. Most people find that a retreat is an opportunity to connect in some way with their soul and we all have different ways to do this.

1 You may be a natural contemplative. Some people can easily sit in silence, meditating, praying or just contemplating. If this suits you, you may like to follow a pattern of prayers or times for meditation, perhaps interspersed with quiet reading or listening to music. Perhaps spend some time each day outside appreciating being in nature.

2 Other people are naturally energetic and find sitting still an impossibility. If this is you, focus your energy with a loose programme of yoga or dance (see page 61). Go for long nature hikes. But do aim to spend at least a little time each day keeping still and trying to hear what your body tells you when you actually allow it to rest.

3 If you find it hard to focus, you may want to try activities such as painting, writing or dancing to bring you in touch with your inner self. Creativity can be a delightful way

to open up the soul. Look back over the exercises and suggestions in Chapter 11 for ideas.

4 Many people manage not to think too deeply most of the time by immersing themselves in activities, even if it's just reading a book or listening to music. If you know you are avoiding issues, try to let yourself give up doing; instead, be quiet and contemplative for at least part of your retreat.

5 There may be a particular issue or event you want to focus on during your retreat. This could be a joyful event (conception, a relationship, a career shift) or a sad one (illness, separation or death). Think about the best ways to work with your issue.

6 This could be a good opportunity for trying out ritual or building a shrine, or any of the other ideas in this book.

7 You may want to do absolutely nothing. And that's fine.

Do-it-yourself retreating

Of course, you don't have to go anywhere in order to retreat. Although it is undoubtedly easier to put aside the detritus of everyday life when you are in a different environment, it's not impossible to retreat in the comfort of your own home.

RETREAT WEEKEND Try a retreat weekend to get a feel for this kind of spiritual holiday. You will need to do some preparing, so allow yourself enough time to get ready.

• Warn people that you are going to be on retreat. If you'd rather keep the reason secret, you can make some other excuse, but make it clear that you are effectively out of touch. You might want to disconnect the telephone or put on the answerphone. Put a 'Do not disturb' sign on your door. If you have family or friends who live with you, try to pick a time when they will be away. Don't collect your mail, or leave it unopened.

• Get in all your provisions. Make sure you have all the food, drink, music, books, candles, incense … whatever … that you will need, so that you don't have to make sorties to the outside world for more. Find an attractive storage box in which to keep things, so you can use them whenever you retreat.

• Clean your space physically and cleanse it spiritually (see the space-cleansing exercises on pages 97–8). You might want to dedicate the space for your retreat with a special ritual.

• Think about the energy you want for your retreat. Should it be vibrant and energizing, or calm and relaxing? Does it need to be nurturing and comforting? Bring in whatever you can to help provide the best possible atmosphere.

• Pick out suitable, comfortable clothes – particularly for any activities you are planning. Will you be warm enough if you are sitting meditating? Are your shoes comfortable for long walks? Do you have 'messy' clothes if you're going to paint?

MINI-RETREAT If you can, it's a great idea to incorporate 'mini-retreats' as a regular part of life. You might set aside an afternoon every weekend, or an hour at night, or even just 15 or 20 minutes once in a while. But make it a time that is just for you. Keep a box or drawer full of your retreat 'props': candles, incense, inspirational books and tapes, maybe the tarot or I Ching, drawing or writing materials. Dedicate your retreat time as 'sacred time' with a ritual, such as lighting a candle or burning some aromatherapy oil, and saying a prayer or reciting a poem. You may like to do some smudging or space cleansing to make your space special.

This could be a time just to sit and think, do some painting or writing, or pray or meditate. It might be the time to carry out a long-term project (such as self-therapy). It doesn't matter how you structure it, but do make sure that, for that time, you aren't disturbed and can do as you wish.

Mental retreating

There are times when we all need to 'get away'. You could be in an unpleasant meeting, crammed on a train or stuck in a situation you really dislike. You can't physically get away, but you can take yourself off to a private mental retreat.

1 Take a few slow, deep breaths to calm yourself. Start to focus on your breathing and notice its rhythm.

2 Start breathing into your solar plexus area, visualizing it becoming soft and warm. This, in itself, is very calming.

3 Imagine that the energy in your solar plexus is bubbling up like a spring – it bubbles and bubbles until it bursts into a golden shower of light and energy. This spreads out all around you, settling into an encompassing golden bubble of light.

4 The bubble keeps you safe and relaxed, and protected from any negative impulses or energies around you. If you like, you can call on further images – use any that will help.

5 If you feel that someone wishes you harm, you can slightly modify the bubble. As it extends around you, imagine it forms into a big glass box, the sides of which are made up of gleaming mirrors. Any negative energy that is sent towards you will bounce off the mirrors and be sent back to your aggressor.

19 Death

We all die. It's the one certainty in life. Yet most of us steadfastly refuse to think about death. We shut it out from our consciousness and try to pretend it doesn't exist, that it won't happen if we don't think about it. Why does death frighten us so much?

Maybe it's because death is such an unknown quantity, or perhaps it's because we hate the idea that we could lose our identity, our self. It may be the thought that death means we will lose our material possessions, our loved ones, our consciousness. Some people, on the other hand, are terrified of pain. These are all very real and valid fears, which should not be lightly dismissed. Yet, by turning our backs on death, we do ourselves and our lives a disservice. By looking calmly and clearly at death and what it means, we can, paradoxically, learn a lot about living. Pause right now and ask yourself what your thoughts are concerning death.

- Are you frightened of death? Are you frightened of your own death or that of others'?
- What do you find most frightening?
- Have you experienced the death of anyone close to you? What feelings did it bring up for you?
- Have you ever thought about your own death?
- What words would you use to describe death?
- Is death always a bad thing?
- Do you believe in an afterlife? In reincarnation? Or do you believe that death is the end?

It might be a useful exercise to write out your feelings about death as free-association, or as a poem or a story. Alternatively, you may feel drawn to the idea of painting death or modelling it out of clay. Imagine you were dancing with Death – what would that dance be like? What kind of figure would Death be: would it be the stock image of the Grim Reaper or something different? Spend some time looking at the various images of death in mythologies and religions from around the world. In some, Death is seen as kindly or compassionate, or stern and just. Think about how much your ideas of death are based on society's general avoidance and fear of it – and what you really feel about it when you remove that layer of fear.

Death as a lesson for life

Ask almost anyone who has survived a serious illness or life-threatening accident, or had a near-death experience, and they will all say the same thing: coming close to death made them really appreciate the life that they have and made them determined to live each year, each day, each minute as if it really mattered. I have dear friends who have cancer and say it is the best thing that has ever happened to them, as it has made them realize how incredible life really is and how often and how foolishly we tend to waste it.

We can all learn from that for, if we choose to ignore death, there is nothing to remind us that life is precious. Truly none of us can tell when we will die. The first lesson of death is that we should live our lives as if every minute mattered. We should ensure that our lives have meaning – that, when we do come to die, we can look back over our lives with joy, satisfaction and peace, rather than with regret, anger and sadness.

Imagine that you have been told you have just one year to live then take some time to think about the following questions.

- What would you want to do with that year?
- Are there things that you have always wanted to do, but have put off?
- What job would you really love to have done?
- Are there people you love, but have lost touch with?
- With whom would you spend that year?
- Are there enemies you feel you would like to forgive?
- Is there any unfinished business to which you should attend before dying?

Spend time on this and really think about it. Why wait until you have only a year? Why not put some of your thoughts into practice right now?

Do you hate your job? Change it! Do you have regrets about things you never tried? Try them. Are there people you should be in touch with? Write a letter or ring them. Don't leave any possibility of regret in your life. Forgive any old enemies – it's not worth the energy of holding on to hate.

If you like, you can take this exercise even further. Imagine that you had only a month, a week, a day, an hour: what would be your priorities? You may be surprised by your answers. Return to this exercise frequently, at the very least once a year, to make sure you keep on track. It's also a great exercise if you tend to project your hopes off into the future: 'I'll be happy when ... I have that new job/bigger house/ideal relationship/perfect body, etc.' We all do it, but focusing on the really important things that are in your life right now can put your life into perspective.

Are you spending too much time on your work and not enough with your children? Do you take your partner, your parents, your friends for granted? Are you resisting enjoying life because you're waiting to lose a few pounds? Don't wait too long – it may be too late.

What is death?

Do you remember the time before you were born? It's highly unlikely. Death is simply a transition, like birth, from one existence to another. Tibetan Buddhism has charted the terrain of death to a degree unsurpassed by any other religion and it has a lot to teach us. According to the Tibetans, there are actually six principal *bardos*, or transition periods:

- Life
- Sleep and dreaming
- Meditation
- Dying
- Intrinsic radiance
- Becoming or rebirth

In fact, we spend our entire lives moving through transitions. If you think about it, there are constant small births and deaths: the start or end of a relationship; leaving an old job and starting a new one; the welcoming into the family of a child or pet; the onset and end of illness; and so on. Nature provides us with the perfect model: the year moves through change from fresh beginnings to ripeness to decay and finally death. Then the whole wonderful cycle begins again. If we see that life is an endless cycle of birth, maturation, death and rebirth, it gives us the sense that our lives are not finite.

It pays to look on the *bardos* as moments of opportunity and potential – at every point of transition we have the precious opportunity of change. We can transform ourselves as often as we wish. Every night you go to sleep as one person and wake up another: take advantage of that.

Who are you?

The one vital lesson we all need to learn is to discover our true selves, to balance our inner natures. You will, I hope, be far closer to an understanding of yourself if you have worked through many of the exercises in this book. In particular, take time to look deeply at your relationships and heal any that are painful or unpleasant. If you find this hard, it might be worth looking into some form of psychotherapy or practising the empty-chair technique (see page 26) to understand the other person's point of view. Let go of any old griev-ances. Perhaps write letters to people – you don't even have to post them (you may want to have a ritual in which you burn them and release the negativity). On the other hand, it might be very healing to send them!

Meditation is an incredibly useful tool in gaining self-understanding and acceptance: notice that it is one of the Tibetan bardos in its own right. Make the time to practise the meditation exercises in Chapter 2. In addition, you may like to introduce a life-enhancing practice known as *Tonglen*.

Tonglen is a Buddhist meditation practice that can have remarkable effects on your rela-tionships and your entire life. It is a powerful way to rid yourself of any negative and toxic emotions that may be clogging your soul – such as anger, jealousy, hate and fear.

- Sit comfortably either on a chair or on the floor with your back straight (you may wish to sit on a small cushion so that your back naturally becomes aligned).
- Allow yourself to become aware of your breathing. Sit just observing your breath for about 5 minutes or try counting 21 out breaths.
- Now visualize someone you love dearly in front of you. As you breathe in, breathe into yourself any pain, upset and anger they might be feeling. Allow yourself to open up to them totally and without stinting.
- As you breathe out, breathe all that is good in you into them. Imagine their pain and suffering being transformed inside you into healing light – you are not holding their suffering, but instead transforming it.
- Repeat this for around 5 minutes.
- You can repeat this with as many people as you like. Keep practising until you are really proficient and can feel the healing energy inside you at will.

When you have perfected this exercise, you are ready for the next step. Instead of someone you love, imagine someone you dislike or even hate in front of you. Now trans-form their pain and anger, and give them back the pure, healing light of love. You may baulk at this, but stick with it. Once you can perform Tonglen in this way for your greatest enemies, you will have taken a huge step forwards in your soul development. You may also see that this exercise will have a noticeable effect on the disliked person or people. Expect surprises!

Now you have reached the end of this book, you will, I hope, hold fresh insights and be a different person from the one who started it. You might choose to go back and work more with the material or you may be ready to read another book and learn more in a different way. I think the same is true of life and death. You may come back and learn more here in this world – or you may go elsewhere. But the journey remains and I hope yours is filled with wonder and deep joy.

Further Reading

PART ONE

ART THERAPY
Brown, Daniel, *Art Therapies*, London, Thorsons, 1997

COLOUR THERAPY
Gimbel, Theo, *Healing with Colour*, London, Gaia, 1994

DREAMS
Weiss, Lillie, *Practical Dreaming*, Oakland CA, New Harbinger Publications, 1999

FAMILY
Bryan, Mark, *Codes of Love*, London, Simon & Schuster, 1999

FENG SHUI
Kingston, Karen, Clear your *Clutter with Feng Shui, London*, Piatkus, 1998
Rossbach, Sarah, *Interior Design with Feng Shui*, London, Rider, 1987
Spear, William, *Feng Shui made Easy*, London, Thorsons, 1995

FLOATING
Hutchison, Michael, *The Book of Floating*, New York, Quill, 1984

FLOWER AND GEM THERAPY
Harvey, Clare G and Cochrane, Amanda, *The Encyclopaedia of Flower Remedies*, London, Thorsons, 1995

LIGHT THERAPY
Liberman, Jacob, *Light – Medicine of the Future*, Santa Fé, Bear & Company, 1991

MEDITATION
Strand, Clark, *The Wooden Bowl*, Dublin, Newleaf, 1999

METAMORPHIC TECHNIQUE
Saint-Pierre, Gaston and Shapiro, Debbie, *The Metamorphic Technique*, Shaftesbury, Element, 1982

MINDFULNESS
Kabat-Zinn, Jon, *Mindfulness Meditation for Everyday Life*, London, Piatkus, 1994

NLP
O'Connor, Joseph and McDermott, Ian, *NLP*, London, Thorsons, 1996

REIKI
The Reiki Alliance, 27 Lavington Road, London W13 9NN (020 8579 3813) www.reikialliance.org.uk

RELATIONSHIPS
Davies, Dr Brenda, *Affairs of the Heart*, London, Hodder & Stoughton, 2000

SEXUALITY
Richardson, Diana, *The Love Keys*, Shaftesbury, Element, 1999

SOUND HEALING
D'Angelo, James, *Healing with the Voice*, London, Thorsons, 2000
Goldman, Jonathan, *Healing Sounds*, Shaftesbury, Element, 1992

STRESS
Adams, Jenni, *Stress a Friend for Life*, Saffron Walden, C W Daniel, 1998

TALKING THERAPIES
Avery, Brice, *Psychotherapy*, London, Thorsons, 1996

WORK
Williams, Nick, *The Work we were Born to Do*, Shaftesbury, Element, 1999

WRITING
Schneider, Myra and Killick, John, *Writing for Self-Discovery*, Shaftesbury, Element, 1998

VASTU SHASTRA
Niranjan Babu, B., *Handbook of Vastu*, New Delhi, UBSPD, 1997

PART TWO

DEATH
Levine, Stephen, *A Year to Live*, London, Thorsons, 1997

PRAYER
Weston, Walter, *How Prayer Heals*, Charlottesville, Hampton Roads, 1998

RETREATING
Louden, Jennifer, *The Woman's Retreat Book*, New York, HarperSanFrancisco, 1997

RITUAL
Alexander, Jane, *Sacred Rituals at Home*, New York, Sterling, 2000

SACRED SPACE
Alexander, Jane, *Spirit of the Home*, London, Thorsons, 1998

SHAMANISM
Rutherford, Leo, *Shamanism*, London, Thorsons, 1996

SHRINES AND ALTARS
Linn, Denise, *Altars*, London, Ebury Press, 1999
Streep, Peg, *Altars Made Easy*, New York, HarperCollins, 1997

SPACE CLEARING
Linn, Denise, *Space Clearing*, London, Ebury Press, 2000

SMUDGING
Alexander, Jane, *The Smudge Pack*, London, Thorsons, 1999

SPIRITUAL TRADITIONS
Freke, Timothy, *Encyclopedia of Spirituality*, New Alresford, Godsfield, 2000

Resources

When writing to organizations please include a large SAE. Many websites now have on-line registers of practitioners, so checking the website first. All information is correct at the time of going to print but organizations do change address so our apologies if any become out of date.

UK

PART ONE

ART THERAPY
British Association of Art Therapists, Mary Ward House, 5 Tavistock Place, London W1H 9SN (020 7383 3774) www.baat.co.uk

AUTOGENIC TRAINING
British Autogenic Society (BAS), Royal London Homoeopathic Hospital, Great Ormond Street, London WC1N 3HR
www.autogenic-therapy.org.uk

DANCE THERAPY
Biodanza UK, 48 Clifford Avenue, London SW14 7BP (020 8392 1433) Email martello@biodanza.demon.co.uk

DREAMS
Many Jungian psychotherapists use dreams as part of their work.
The Association of Jungian Analysts, 7 Eton Avenue, London NW3 3EL (020 7794 8711)

FLOATING
The Floatation Tank Association, PO Box 11024, London SW4 7ZF (020 7627 4962)
www.floatationtankassociation.net

MEDITATION
There are around 60 UK centers teaching Transcendental Meditation.
For details contact 0990 143733
www.transcendental-meditation.org.uk

NLP
Association of Neuro-Linguistic Programming, PO Box 78, Stourbridge, DY8 4ZJ (01785 660665) www.anlp.org

SOLUTION-FOCUSED THERAPY
see *United Kingdom Council for Psychotherapy* (Talking therapies, below)

TALKING THERAPIES
United Kingdom Council for Psychotherapy, 167–9 Great Portland Street, London W1W 5PF (020 7436 3002)
www.psychotherapy.org.uk

TIMELINE THERAPY
The Institute of Human Development, Freepost, Tonbridge, Kent TN11 8BR (01732 834354).

PART TWO

RETREATING
The Retreat Company, The Manor House, Kings Norton, Leicestershire, LE7 9BA (0116 2599211) www.retreat-co.co.uk

SHAMANISM

Eagle's Wing, 58 Westbere Road, London NW2 3RU (020 7435 8174) www.shamanism.co.uk

The Sacred Trust, PO Box 16, Uckfield, East Sussex TN22 5WD (01825 840574) www.sacredtrust.org

SMUDGING

see Shamanism, above

SPACE CLEARING

Karen Kingston, Suite 401, Langham House, 24 Margaret Street, London W1N 7LB (07000 772232) www.spaceclearing.com Workshops and products.

USA

PART ONE

ART THERAPY

American Art Therapy Association, 1202 Allanson Road, Mundelein, IL 60060 (1 888 290 0878 or 847 949 6064; fax 847 566 4580) Email arttherapy@ntr.net www.arttherapy.org/ss

DANCE THERAPY

American Dance Therapy Association, TDTA National Office, business hours 8:30am–4:00pm (410 997 4040; fax 4l0 997 4048) Email info@adta.org www.adta.org

DREAM THERAPY

The Association for the Study of Dreams, PO Box 1166, Orinda, CA 94563 (925 258 1822; fax 925 258 1821) Email asdreams@aol.com www.asdreams.org

MEDITATION

Holistic-online.com, Email info@holisticonline.com www.holistic-online.com/stress/stress_autogenic-training.htm

International Meditation Center, 4920 Rose Drive, Westminster MD 21158 (410 346 7889; fax 410 346 7133) ccpl.carr.org/~imcusa/

A practical guide to autogenetic training On-line course published by published by HSCTI, PO Box 1298, Woodstock, GA 30188 www.magitech.com/autogenic

NEUROTHERAPY

The Neuro-Linguistic Programming Information Center, www.nlpinfo.com

The Society of Neuro-Linguistic Programming, John La Valle, President, Box 424, Hopatcong, NJ 07843 (201 770 3600; fax 201 770 0314)

SOLUTION-FOCUSED THERAPY

American Counseling Association, 5999 Stevenson Avenue, Alexandria, VA 22304 (703 823 9800; fax 703 823 0252) www.counseling.org

SPA THERAPY

Floatspa.com, Lighthouse Point, Florida (954 899 6182) Email info@floatspa.com www.floatspa.com

PART TWO

RETREATING

Body/Mind Restoration Retreats, 56 Lieb Road, Spencer, NY 14883 (607 272 0694) www.bodymindretreats.com

Index

Acknowledgements

This is a book I could never have written single-handedly – so I would like to give heart-felt thanks to the many experts who have given so generously their time and knowledge to me. They include: Angela Hope-Murray, Judith Morrison, Doja Purkitt, Dr Rajendra Sharma, Andrew Johnson, Ruth Delman and Kenneth Gibbons, Dr Tamara Voronina, Roger Newman Turner, Dr Andrew Lockie, Roger Savage, Penelope Ritchie, Keith and Chrissie Mason, Kate Roddick, Rosalie Samet, Dr Natsagdorj, Karin Weisensel, Dr Mohammad Salim Khan, Linda Lazarides, Patrick Holford, Dr Marilyn Glenville, Fiona Arrigo, Nicola Griffin, Andrew Chevalier, Christine Steward, Godfrey Devereux, Sebastian Pole, Charlotte Katz, Sue Weston, Malcolm Kirsch, Joel Carbonnel, Kate Kelly, Gail Barlow, Barbara McCrea, Julie Crocker, Jane Thurnell-Read, Geraint and Sylvia Jones-David, Wilma Tait, Tom Williams, Sarah Shurety, Liz Williams, Simon Brown, William Spear, Karen Kingston, Denise Linn, Gina Lazenby, Kajal Sheth, Lynne Crawford, Rob Russell, Kati Cottrell-Blanc, Jane Mayers, Richard Lanham, Ron Wilgosh, Dave Hawkes, Jo Hogg, Kieran Foley, Jennie Crewdson, Terry Peterson, Allan Rudolf, Carol Logan, Tony Bailey, Angela Renton, Gillie Gilbert, Sarah Dening, Patricia Martello, Gabrielle Roth, Caroline Born, Shan, Leo Rutherford, Kenneth Meadows, Howard Charing, William Bloom, Will Parfitt, Vera Diamond, Maria Mercati, Julian Baker, Monica Anthony, Phil Parker, Jon Mason, Jeff Leonard, Peter Bartlett, Corina Petter, Sue Ricks, Pat Morrell, Rosalyn Journeaux, Elaine Arthey, Pim de Gryff, Sara Hooley, Eileen Fairbane, Dee Jones, Jessica Loeb, Emma Field, Narendra Mehta, Jill Dunley, Agni Eckroyd, Harry Oldfield, Rosamund Webster, Margaret-Anne Pauffley and Paul Dennis, Natalie Handley, Chris James, Susan Lever, Angelika Hochadel, Gaston Saint-Pierre.

Lots of love to the original Williams family who started me off on this curious path and to the many friends and fellow seekers who have guided me along the way.

A large debt of gratitude to Bonnie Estridge who introduced me to Carlton Books and to everyone there.

A big hug as always to über-agent Judy Chilcote.